Palgrave Studies in Masculinity, Sport and Exercise

Series Editors

Rory Magrath
Solent University
Southampton, UK

Jamie Cleland
University of South Australia
Adelaide, Australia

Eric Anderson
University of Winchester
Winchester, UK

Recent years have seen the emergence of a considerable body of research investigating the complex nature of masculinity, and how it impacts on a wide-range of sporting (and exercise) cultures. Palgrave Studies in Masculinity, Sport and Exercise is the first series solely dedicated to providing innovative and high-quality scholarship within this area of study. The series welcomes proposals for research monographs, Palgrave Pivots and edited collections examining critical, empirical and theoretical issues related to the study of masculinity, sport and exercise. The series has an international focus – both in terms of its authorship and readership – and welcomes relevant scholarship by established and emerging scholars in the field from any country.

James Alder

Military Men, Physical Exercise, and Post-Traumatic Stress Disorder

palgrave
macmillan

James Alder
University of Winchester
Winchester, UK

ISSN 2662-740X ISSN 2662-7418 (electronic)
Palgrave Studies in Masculinity, Sport and Exercise
ISBN 978-3-032-08956-4 ISBN 978-3-032-08957-1 (eBook)
https://doi.org/10.1007/978-3-032-08957-1

Cover credit: Svetlana Isochenko / Alamy

This Palgrave Macmillan imprint is published by the registered company Springer Nature Switzerland AG.
The registered company address is: Gewerbestrasse 11, 6330 Cham, Switzerland

Dedication

To all military servicemen and veterans who carry the unseen weight of PTSD. Your resilience in the face of invisible wounds, and your courage to keep going, even when words fail, have shaped every page of this work.

To the loved ones who stand beside you in the shadows, bearing the silence, the setbacks, and the daily unknowns with grace and unwavering loyalty.

Your battles are real. Your strength is undeniable.

This book is for you.

Preface

This monograph explores the interwoven themes of military masculinities, physical exercise, and post-traumatic stress disorder (PTSD), drawing on empirical evidence and my lived experience as both a veteran and academic. By integrating personal narrative with qualitative and quantitative methodologies, the work offers a multifaceted analysis of trauma and recovery within military and veteran contexts. Central to this exploration is the role of masculinity, cultural scripts, and embodied approaches in shaping the recovery process.

The structure of the book is designed to progress logically from context and theory to personal narrative and applied research:

Chapter 1 lays the groundwork by outlining the clinical and historical context of PTSD in military men. It introduces symptomology, diagnostic evolution, and the gendered dynamics that shape help-seeking behaviours.

Chapter 2 delves deeper into these themes by analysing how masculinities influence symptom expression and treatment engagement. It provides a critical overview of therapeutic modalities and highlights barriers linked to hegemonic masculine ideals.

Chapter 3 expands the analysis by focusing on the role of the body in trauma recovery. It argues that physical exercise can serve as a culturally congruent and accessible form of intervention, particularly for those socialised within hypermasculine military environments.

Chapter 4 presents an autoethnographic account of my own recovery journey through CrossFit. This chapter offers a reflexive and personal narrative that connects embodied healing to broader cultural and psychological frameworks.

Chapter 5 presents findings from a qualitative study examining how military veterans engage with physical activity as a therapeutic strategy for managing PTSD. It explores themes of identity, discipline, social belonging, and emotional regulation through exercise.

Chapter 6 reports the results of a quantitative investigation into the effects of structured physical exercise on PTSD symptom reduction. This chapter provides statistical evidence to support claims made in earlier narrative and qualitative sections.

Chapter 7 synthesises the findings and draws out the practical, clinical, and policy-related implications of the research. It also offers recommendations for future directions in trauma recovery, especially those that engage with culturally resonant practices.

The book concludes with a comprehensive Bibliography and Index, alongside additional front matter including a List of Abbreviations and Tables, as well as statements on Ethics Approval and Competing Interests.

Methodology is woven throughout the chapters rather than presented in isolation. This integrated approach reflects the complex and multifaceted nature of the inquiry, combining autoethnographic, qualitative, and quantitative methods. By embedding methodology within relevant chapters, the monograph maintains narrative continuity and contextual depth while meeting scholarly standards.

Ultimately, this work aims to contribute to evolving conversations around PTSD, masculinity, and embodied recovery. It seeks to influence how trauma is conceptualised and addressed by offering both academic rigour and experiential insight grounded in the lived realities of veterans.

Winchester, UK James Alder

Acknowledgements

I would like to express my sincere thanks to the military veteran charities Combat Stress and Help for Heroes for their generous support of this research. Their ongoing commitment to improving the mental health of veterans remains vital, and their encouragement of this project has been deeply appreciated.

I am especially grateful to CrossFit® for granting permission to use their brand name throughout this research and for supporting the auto-ethnographic component exploring PTSD recovery through structured physical activity. I wish to thank Anthony Mosher, who designed my CrossFit® Programme and mentored me during my recovery. I also extend my thanks to Dave MacDougal and the staff at CrossFit Basinview CFB, as well as the CrossFit® community at CFB Halifax, whose support and camaraderie sustained me throughout the process.

I am indebted to Eric Anderson, John Batten, and Jo Batey for their academic guidance and support. Their insights and encouragement played a pivotal role in shaping this work, and their collegiality has been a source of personal and professional strength.

My heartfelt thanks goes to my partner, Raeanne Fletcher, for her unwavering love, patience, and encouragement throughout this academic journey. Her understanding gave me the space to think and write, while her support helped bring this work to completion. I also wish to acknowledge my children, whose patience and encouragement provided balance and inspiration throughout this process.

Finally, I am deeply grateful to all the veterans who participated in this Chapter. Your willingness to share your experiences and place your trust in this research is sincerely appreciated. Your strength and openness have made this work possible, and your contributions will help inform better support for others navigating similar challenges.

Competing Interests The author declares that there are no competing financial, professional, or personal interests that have influenced the research, writing, or content of this monograph.

Ethics Approval Ethical approval for the research presented in this monograph was granted by the University of Winchester Ethics Committee. All research involving human participants was conducted in accordance with institutional guidelines and ethical standards. Informed consent was obtained from all participants, and appropriate measures were taken to ensure confidentiality, voluntary participation, and the right to withdraw at any stage.

Competing Interests The author has no competing interests to declare that are relevant to the content of this manuscript.

About the Book

"Military Men, Physical Exercise, and Post-Traumatic Stress Disorder" offers an interdisciplinary examination of how structured physical activity may function as a meaningful and culturally appropriate intervention for military veterans living with post-traumatic stress disorder (PTSD). Drawing on the author's personal experience as a British Army veteran and Chartered Psychologist, the monograph integrates autoethnographic reflection, qualitative research, and quantitative analysis to provide a multidimensional understanding of trauma recovery.

The book is framed by an exploration of the cultural and institutional expectations placed upon military men, particularly those associated with hegemonic forms of masculinity. Traits such as emotional control, stoicism, and physical endurance are frequently valorised in military contexts, yet these same attributes can inhibit help-seeking and increase psychological vulnerability following exposure to trauma. The monograph critically interrogates how these gendered norms shape both the manifestation of PTSD and the reception of conventional mental health interventions.

Physical exercise is positioned not only as a physiological tool for improving mental health, but also as a culturally resonant practice through which veterans may begin to reconstruct a sense of agency, identity, and belonging. Activities such as CrossFit®, and other group-based, performance-oriented forms of exercise, are examined as potential spaces where therapeutic engagement can occur in ways that align with, rather than oppose, the participants' existing values and identities. The book carefully considers both the potential benefits and risks of aligning recovery with masculine-coded practices, emphasising the importance of trauma-informed, identity-sensitive approaches.

This volume contributes to current debates across psychology, sport and exercise science, trauma studies, and military and masculinity research. It will be of interest to academics, practitioners, veteran support organisations, and policymakers seeking to develop holistic, contextually relevant interventions for trauma recovery. The monograph combines scholarly analysis with lived experience to offer a distinctive and timely contribution to the evolving discourse on mental health support for military veterans.

Contents

About the Author

James Alder is a lecturer and researcher at Arden University and a Chartered Psychologist with the British Psychological Society. His work explores the transformative potential of physical activity in the treatment of post-traumatic stress disorder (PTSD). His research focuses on exercise as a culturally meaningful and holistic intervention, particularly for individuals from military backgrounds. Drawing on lived experience, his work critically engages with the intersections of masculinity, identity, and trauma recovery.

James Alder's research agenda centres on non-traditional, embodied approaches to psychological healing. He investigates how structured physical activity can restore autonomy, competence, and relatedness in those living with PTSD, positioning exercise not merely as rehabilitation but as a pathway to reclaiming selfhood. His scholarship employs both narrative and empirical methods, using autoethnography, qualitative interviews, and applied sport psychology to examine the role of movement, discipline, and community in recovery.

This monograph brings together James Alder's personal insights and research expertise to challenge prevailing models of PTSD treatment. By weaving reflective narrative with evidence-based analysis, it aims to reshape how trauma is understood and addressed, especially among military men, and offers valuable perspectives for scholars, clinicians, and support organisations alike.

Abbreviations

APA	American Psychological Association
ATP-CPT	Adapted Trauma-Focused Cognitive Processing Therapy
BPS	British Psychological Society
CBT	Cognitive Behavioural Therapy
CF	CrossFit®
CFB	Canadian Forces Base
CFT	Compassion-Focused Therapy
CNS	Central Nervous System
CPT	Cognitive Processing Therapy
CS	Combat Stress
DSM-5	Diagnostic and Statistical Manual of Mental Disorders, Fifth Edition
EMDR	Eye Movement Desensitisation and Reprocessing
FITT	Frequency, Intensity, Time, and Type
GAD	Generalised Anxiety Disorder
GIP	Guaranteed Income Payment
GP	General Practitioner
HIIT	High-Intensity Interval Training
H4H	Help for Heroes
HR	Heart Rate
HRV	Heart Rate Variability
ICD	International Classification of Diseases
ICD-11	International Classification of Diseases, 11th Revision
LSD	Long Slow Distance (aerobic endurance training)
MBSR	Mindfulness-Based Stress Reduction
MDD	Major Depressive Disorder
METs	Metabolic Equivalents
MH	Mental Health

MIRT	Multimodal Intervention Rehabilitation Therapy
MOD	Ministry of Defence
MOI	Mechanism of Injury
MRSA	Methicillin-Resistant Staphylococcus Aureus
MST	Military Sexual Trauma
MVPA	Moderate to Vigorous Physical Activity
NHS	National Health Service
OCD	Obsessive Compulsive Disorder
PCL-5	PTSD Checklist for DSM-5
PE	Prolonged Exposure / Prolonged Exposure Therapy
PFA	Psychological First Aid
PFT	Physical Fitness Test
PNS	Peripheral Nervous System / Parasympathetic Nervous System
PRT	Progressive Resistance Training
PT	Physical Training / Personal Trainer
PTSD	Post-Traumatic Stress Disorder
QoL	Quality of Life
RCT	Randomised Controlled Trial
RPE	Rate of Perceived Exertion
RPM	Revolutions/Repetitions per Minute (context-dependent)
RT	Resistance Training
S&C	Strength and Conditioning
SDT	Self-Determination Theory
SNRI	Serotonin–Norepinephrine Reuptake Inhibitor
SSRI	Selective Serotonin Reuptake Inhibitor
TBI	Traumatic Brain Injury
TMS	Transcranial Magnetic Stimulation
TRX	Total Resistance Exercise
VA	Veterans Affairs (US)
VAMs	Visual Analogue Measures
VBT	Velocity-Based Training
VO2 max	Maximal Oxygen Uptake
WHO	World Health Organization
WOD	Workout of the Day (CrossFit term)
ZTT	Zero-Tolerance Training (behavioural regimes)

List of Tables

CHAPTER 1

Understanding PTSD in Military Men

My Soldiering Journey

I grew up in the post-industrial town of Wigan, where career opportunities open to me were few. I came from a white, working-class family which consisted of an Irish father (Council highway maintenance worker) and English mother (housewife). I was the eldest of four children: two sons and two daughters. I had always found the military very appealing. This interest started when my uncle William told me stories of his experiences of serving in the British Army. The excitement I felt on hearing my uncle's tales of far and distant countries that he explored alongside the pride I felt in him for protecting our national security, provided me the incentive to pursue a military career.

In 1989, aged 16 and waiting to take my GCSE Exams, I started the process of joining the British Army. It was a lengthy process, with an initial interview and eligibility assessment at the Army careers office in Wigan. After two weeks, I was informed that I had passed all of the enlistment criteria. The next step was to travel to the Army careers office in Manchester to attend the medical examination. This medical was very thorough, including my first experience of the "cough and drop" examination (we would drop our shorts and cough, while the doctor examined our testicles). This was the first time I had been naked in front of a female doctor.

J. Alder, *Military Men, Physical Exercise, and Post-Traumatic Stress Disorder*, Palgrave Studies in Masculinity, Sport and Exercise, https://doi.org/10.1007/978-3-032-08957-1_1

I was suffering from the flu during this medical, which affected my hearing. I therefore failed the hearing exam. I thus had to cough and drop twice: fortunately, passing the second time. I was now cleared to proceed to the Army selection centre, in Sutton Coldfield. The selection centre examined recruits across two areas: fitness and psychological aptitude. Being at the selection centre also provided me with a taste of life inside a military camp and some insight into what would be expected of me if I were to become a soldier.

The fitness tests consisted of a one-and-a-half mile run as a squad followed by one-and-a-half-mile individual run, which had to be completed in under ten minutes and thirty seconds. Sit-ups and pull-ups followed the run and were marked on a sliding scale dependent on the service into which you were enlisting. It was a very challenging experience due to dealing with meeting new people in unfamiliar surroundings, plus the pressure of the fitness assessment and uncertainty about the results.

Following the fitness test, I waited to see if I had met the criteria to become a soldier. When I was informed that I was successful and was being offered a place in the British Army, the sense of achievement was almost overwhelming. Having not experienced what success felt like after struggling to find my way through my childhood. I was overcome with raw emotion. Tears followed by smiles. I had overcome the selection criteria and gained a place in the Army.

Finally, I attended the Manchester Army Careers office and had to recite my "oath of allegiance" in front of a colonel from the British Army. It was the most nervous I had ever been. This made me a soldier, at least on paper. I received my first days' pay of eight pounds sterling. At that time, as a teenager, this was a lot of money.

The next few months consisted of my final days attending classes at secondary school and taking my GCSE exams. It was challenging trying to maintain my focus and pass my exams while awaiting my date of enlistment to start my basic training. However, I was very fortunate within my group of friends, as I was a 16-year-old who had already found work, which was the cause of much anxiety throughout my peer groups. Nevertheless, the whole period was frustrating. Still, as the eldest child I was expected to remain a role model for my siblings and continue a sense of normality. It had not yet occurred to me that I was leaving my family and what impact it might have on them. Instead, I was focused on myself and the new adventure that I had been dreaming about. It was May, and I was waiting to take my last exam when the news finally came. I was to begin my basic training in July at JIB Ouston, Albemarle Barracks in Newcastle upon Tyne (the northeast of England).

On Sunday, 16th July 1989, the day had finally come for me to leave my family and start my journey of becoming a soldier. It all began with my family and I standing at Oxford Road railway station, Manchester, waiting for the train. It was a sunny day, and I was smartly dressed. I had a sense of nervous excitement for the trip ahead but also a sense of fear that I was leaving family and the only security I had ever known.

I arrived at Newcastle upon Tyne, to a towering figure awaiting us on the platform. He was barking out orders for any recruits to follow him outside and board the bus to Albemarle Barracks. Guards carried rifles and squads of soldiers marched and ran around the camp. I was sized-up and issued with all of my military uniform, followed by being run around camp to familiarise me with my new surroundings. I was issued with my regimental number, 24870280. This number would stay with me for my entire military career and would establish both my bureaucratic military identity, and my personal identity transformation as well. The morning routine resembled the start of a formula one race. Alarm bells signalled the beginning of the chaos as the noise of many men running around trying to wash, clean the accommodation and eat breakfast filled my ears. This was all before the daily training programme had even started.

My upbringing with an Irish father had introduced me to the importance of discipline; however, the army discipline was like something I had never experienced before. It was incorporated in every aspect of daily routine and would help to reshape my future behaviours and mould me into a soldier. All the skills I would require to be able to manage the challenges of being a soldier in the British Army and survive in battle would be taught to me in the next eleven months.

The process was not a smooth transition. My previous self was stripped back. I was to relinquish all elements of individual thought, opinions, and views of the world, so that the body and mind were able to accept the new information to become the end product: a soldier.

Early memories of my first platoon fitness runs are of shock and pride. The speed we had to maintain while still maintaining our platoon formation was extremely challenging. However, after initial struggles with the pace of the run and running in boots, I was amazed and proud to have made it to the end. Similarly, the first individual run was extraordinarily intense and high paced, which opened my eyes to how army training was going to get me in physical shape like never before.

The fitness-training Programme was progressive and designed to push your endurance. It included weighted platoon runs (running with back-packs weighting 20lb), circuit training, and assault course sessions. Every day I noticed the transition my body and mind were going through. Once physically unfit my body became more athletic, physically and more physically and mentally robust.

The whirlwind of the first three months challenged my ability to keep track of time, moving from bed, drill square, chemical training chamber, running around camp, and learning to fire a rifle. The speed and delivery of military training were exhausting, which gave little time to relax until everyone had finished preparing their kit for the next day.

My first experience using a rifle was a steep learning curve, but we all slowly became confident and proficient enough to proceed to the ranges. The conversations in the barrack-room were all about firing the rifle in the barrack rooms. We were full with bullish confidence about who would be best. However, I felt the nerves and anticipation of the upcoming range day. The big day arrived, and standing waiting to fire my rifle on the 25-metre range was nerve-racking, the loud noise of gunfire filled the air. Dressed in combat uniform, my webbing, body armour, and helmet with my ear defenders covering my ears I heard the commands, “Prone position down”, “Load”, “Fire”. The first press of the trigger.

No other noise other than a dull crack of the hammer striking the round and thump of the bullet hitting the target. I enjoyed firing my rifle, but I was extremely nervous about my evaluation by the platoon sergeant. What I did not know at this point was how necessary this training would be for my tour of Iraq, where the volleys of fire were very real and much louder than firing in the relative safety of the range.

I had minimal life experiences or sense of achievement before joining the Army. However, after a period of hard work, determination and long days of military training, I had earned the right to wear my regimental cap badge. I was now a junior leader in the Queen’s Lancashire Regiment. I was still a long way from finishing training, but I had passed my drill test, map reading, and spent nights under the stars during my first field exercise. During my army training, I had suffered with low confidence and self-esteem due to periods of homesickness and injuries. However, marching around camp wearing my regimental cap badge gave me a great sense of pride and confidence in what I was about to face. Now at the halfway point, we had been awarded weekend passes to leave camp. Therefore, we could enjoy a well-deserved break before continuing with training. The final few months flew by with all our focus on passing the last exercise and the big pass out parade. The final exercise, called the "Final fling" was two weeks of showing off our skills in the field, which resulted in us winning the best platoon award. The build-up for the pass out parade was made up of very long nights on the drill square and marching endlessly around camp until we knew the routine perfectly. The final day had arrived, the sun was shining and there was not a cloud in the sky as we marched towards the parade square. Due to five platoons, being on parade, it was at the time the most significant pass out parade in Albemarle Barracks' recent history. Soldiers within all five platoons were beaming with confidence, showing off all the skills acquired over the past eleven months. Inspections and awards were presented. Our families patiently waited to see us and show their appreciation with cheers and loud applause. The parade marched off the square, and basic training had been completed. I arrived as a boy, but after eleven months of hard work, I had grown into a man.

Regimental Duty

Following basic training, I was assigned to the First Battalion the Queen's Lancashire Regiment and arrived at Weeton Camp for my first day of regimental duty in June 1990. When I turned 18, I was eligible to deploy with my rifle company to Northern Ireland. We flew by Chinook helicopter and landed in Cookstown. I quickly found my feet and became familiar with my new surroundings. The tour lasted six weeks and would be one of many tours of Northern Ireland with time spent patrolling in Cookstown, Dungannon, Pomeroy, and Armagh City from 1991 to 1992. My time in Northern Ireland was different with each tour, due to the change in location.

The majority of my time on patrol was in the countryside and towns of East Tyrone, which provided its own unique challenges. However, when we arrived in Armagh City our area of responsibility increased and so did our workload.

Each time I returned from Northern Ireland, I would grow as a person, and my family noticed the changes when I came home. I was no longer the young man my family recognised. The time spent patrolling the streets of Northern Ireland matured me as a man. Specifically, experience gained in being confronted by hostility from many of the local Catholic population created a steely mental fortitude. After experiencing shots being fired while on patrol, a dramatic rise in heartbeat, and adrenaline would shoot through my body, which fuelled my anger. The camp became our base of security, but the protection it would provide came under threat from gunfire and mortar threats, petrol bombs, abuse from local Catholic populations, and stress from working under fatigue.

The Northern Ireland tour provided multiple exposures to distressing events due to the hostile environment I patrolled. The threatening encounters experienced on patrols brought countless sleepless nights. The ever-increasing threat assessment would put my mind to a heightened state of alertness, due to the increased risk to life. The experiences I encountered patrolling in Northern Ireland helped me to establish both a calmness of my heart and greater cognitive coping strategies for future military combat tours.

In March 1992, we finished our commitment as the provincial rural battalion in Northern Ireland and moved back to our home base to prepare for our next posting. The regiment moved to Wavell Barracks, Berlin, Germany, in April 1992 where our working environment completely changed. Instead of patrolling, we would be conducting field training exercises, which consisted of forced incursion marches carrying our full equipment, rifle range and platoon fighting patrols to prepare for possible deployments.

Once work was done for the day, we would be out enjoying the fruits of our labour. It was "party time", and soldiers knew how to enjoy life. Being in Berlin was a great experience and helped to shape my future career path. In 1993, I would complete my physical training instructors (PTI) course, which set me on a very successful career and allowed me to provide fitness training for my rifle company in British Army Training Unit Suffield (Batus), Canada, and Italy.

I left Germany in 1994, as part of the last British Army regiment to serve in Berlin, and we moved to take up our new home at Bhurtpore Barracks in Tidworth, England. After a short period of 18 months in Tidworth, I moved to Fulwood Barracks, Preston in 1995. My role provided physical training supervision during military formalisation training for potential new Army recruits. The opportunity to have worked in the training and recruitment environment provided a great experience and helped to develop my teaching ability. In December 1998, I finished my time in Preston and was posted to St Lucia Barracks, Omagh, Northern Ireland.

I returned to my regiment in Omagh, Northern Ireland. I found them providing much needed support within the local communities due to the devastation caused by the bombing in Omagh town centre. Northern Ireland had been experiencing a period of peace, when in August 1998, the terrorist organisation, the Real Irish Republican Army, had detonated a car bomb in the town centre of Omagh, that caused destruction and the loss of 29 lives. My regiment had been impacted deeply due to this traumatic event, with many soldiers involved in the clean-up of the scene of the explosion and the setting up of the bubble gymnasium as the scene recovery area. The experiences and emotions shared while working under these extremely distressing conditions helped to solidify the bond between officers and soldiers.

I found myself as a physical training instructor in Omagh and was quickly back into the pace of conducting regimental duty, maintain the soldiers combat fitness levels. Time passed quickly, and my regiment provided security during the annual orange order marching parades in the area, so day-to-day activities would not be disrupted.

During my tour in Omagh, I had decided it was the right time to change my role within my regiment, join a rifle company once again, and follow a mainstream infantry career path. I had worked in the gymnasium for over six years and to gain promotion I would need to leave the gym and join a rifle company. In December 1999, I was posted with my regiment to Alma Barracks, Catterick Garrison, North Yorkshire, and into rifle company B. I had the role of platoon sergeant and prepared the rifle platoon for the upcoming field exercises.

However, I also had to qualify to fill the role and worked hard on infantry field tactics. In 2000, I attended the first part of Platoon Sergeant Battle Course (PSBC), which was the mainstream infantry qualification required for me to hold my role and infantry career.

Between 2000 and 2001, my regiment was asked to fill a physical training instructor post in Banja Luka, Bosnia as part of the NATO tactical group. I was the only individual with enough experience in my regiment to fill the position, so I went on tour to Bosnia as a physical training instructor. My role provided training support for British military personnel while on tour in Bosnia.

On completion of my tour in Bosnia, I deployed with my regiment to Bessbrook Mill, Northern Ireland, as a patrol commander and the year ended with the completion of the field, tactics phase Platoon Sergeant Battle Course (PSBC). I had become a fully qualified rifle platoon sergeant in the infantry, which prepared to me to fill my role confidently. During 2005–2006, my regiment moved to Dhekelia Barracks, Cyprus and this would be the final time it would operate as the Queen's Lancashire Regiment before it joined with two other regiments in 2006 to form the Duke of Lancaster's Regiment.

My Iraq Tour (Telic Nine)

I had been on operational tours in Northern Ireland, Bosnia, and Iraq. Each deployment had provided me with many different operational experiences with each country having its own climatic, operational, and traumatic challenges. These military experiences would build and fundamentally go on to shape my character. Northern Ireland had been my introduction to the role of an infantryman during an operational tour.

To survive as an infantryman on patrol you are required to have physical strength and robustness to carry heavy packs on our back, the grit and determination to dig deep and complete tasks when failure seems guaranteed. The strength of character and composure under pressure established a mental toughness for an infantryman to survive while on patrol. At a very young age, to be accepted by my peer group, I had to quickly establish myself, which meant I would need to carry the heavy equipment on patrol.

I grew into my role within the patrol team following a steep learning curve, and the patrols had become less daunting during my tour of Northern Ireland. My tour of Bosnia had been during a period of peace which allowed me to gain thorough knowledge and understanding of the causes of conflicts with many leading to the needless loss of life. Whereas, Iraq had provided me with greater respect for soldiers who had deployed and fought against the enemy during the war in challenging and distressing circumstances.

Each Iraq tour was given a designation, my tour of Iraq was given Telic Nine, and this would go on to change me forever, even when I could not or would not recognise it. Iraq was a country in turmoil with both Sunni and Shia tribes fighting each other for control of the country. My battle group was in the middle, struggling to maintain order and security. My early days in Iraq were designed to help me familiarise myself with the surroundings and acclimatise to the countries' hot and dry climate. With temperatures reaching above 40 degrees Celsius during the hottest times of the day it was decided to conduct the patrolling at night which reduced any risk of heat exposure and improved our operational role.

Patrolling at night gave us an edge over the terrorists due to our night-time viewing equipment, which helped us perform more effectively when responding to enemy attacks.

Equally, it was very evident that work conducted in Iraq was very different to previous operational tours. There was a need to be adaptable on each patrol from providing support and aid to local civilian populations while also being involved in exchanges of gunfire with terrorists. Telic Nine was a very difficult tour with endless combat incidents on patrols which saw the regiment record its highest loss of life during an operational tour with 12 reported killed by Improvised Explosive Devices (IED), gunfire, and sniper fire.

My first patrol was a quiet event but one which would give me a sense of the size of the task that lay ahead. There were two gates, which allowed patrols to leave the camp. The front gate was the quickest way to reach Basra City but it meant having to pass through the city's rubbish tip.

Patrols left camp at night and navigated the main tracks within the rubbish tip area but the stench of burning tyres and rotting rubbish made your eyes water and made it extremely difficult to breathe. My confidence was quickly replaced with feelings of anxiety and nerves. The smell of rotten rubbish and thick smoke from the burning rubbish and tyres took my breath away, and fear of what possibly lay ahead put me on edge. Once through, however, we quickly composed ourselves and established a foothold in Basra City.

Once completed, we would return to base under the blanket of the night sky. In response to our intrusion the terrorist groups would retaliate with indirect mortar fire. The sound of multiple improvised mortars being fired set off our early warning sirens. Commanders told us to "Take Cover" and we scurried to an area offering safe protection but at an audible distance. I recall diving under protective cover wearing my helmet and body armour. My heartbeat almost drowned out the explosions, and I wondered if this would be the night that I wouldn't survive to hear the all-clear alarm.

This nightly routine continued with noise from warning sirens and explosions. The daily routine would consist of eating and sleeping during the day if the alarms and indirect fire would allow, followed by patrolling at night. This routine would repeat.

I had participated on many patrols during my time in Iraq; each exposed me to challenging tasks under the threat of reprisal from the enemy. Furthermore, one patrol saw more gunfire, explosions from indirect mortar fire and improvised explosive devices than I can count or can remember, the aftermath of which deeply affected my mental health. I also lost friends to the flames of war.

On one patrol, I was in the lead vehicle in a convoy of patrol vehicles as we performed road clearance. We reached a road junction on the patrol route onto Basra City, when a loud explosion broke the silence leaving a tank damaged and crew injured.

The atmosphere completely changed. Everyone was on edge. Yet, under pressure to perform the task assigned to us we continued with the patrol. After a slow and cautious drive into Basra, we arrived at our next task of providing overwatch (a location which allowed my vehicle to observe other patrol tasks while also being able to provide support if required). Everyone was alert and scanning for any threats to our vehicle and patrol group.

After two hours, the sun was rising, and locals were going on with their daily lives. My armoured vehicle had been at our checkpoint when the atmosphere of the local population changed. Civilians rapidly disappeared signalling that attacks were imminent.

They hit hard. Intense targeted gunfire from domestic terrorists at multiple locations prompted the commander to order a quick return fire towards the enemy with rapid vehicle movement to disrupt the attack. However, as soon as our response started to limit the enemy threat, a loud explosion followed by black smoke and metal shrapnel filled the sky. A friendly armoured vehicle had been hit by an IED, which had caused multiple injuries to colleagues.

The two incidents caused anger and distress throughout the patrol group, with two colleagues being left with severe brain injuries due to the force from the blast. The remainder of the crew in the vehicle had been left with bangs, cuts and bruises and were in shock, but thankfully, there were no fatalities. However, the incident had left me troubled by my thoughts which drifted between shock about what had happened and concern about the well-being of the soldiers under my command. The heat and dusty climate had intensified my anxiety, but I had to be focused whilst the patrol continued to move to the next checkpoint in the middle of Basra City.

The primary purpose of the patrol was to provide support to a new infantry regiment to perform its task of obtaining intelligence on terrorist activities and the location of one of the foremost terrorist leaders in Basra City. The meeting had been concluded when the patrol command group had been concerned by the build-up of people who had chanted and rioted around the meeting location.

Gunfire from terrorists had dispersed the crowd, with some civilian casualties. Our role had been to provide security during the patrol, when my vehicle became subjected to enemy fire. Under the threat of sniper fire, my armoured vehicle had been attacked by indirect mortar fire with many of the explosions landing all around our patrol holding location. The noise of mortar fire and debris had hit my vehicle, which intensified my sense of anticipation, especially after the previous two incidents during the patrol. Loud bangs of gunfire filled the air and sporadic metal-on-metal pings could be heard as bullets hit the command console turret at the top of my armoured vehicle and the main bodies of our armoured vehicles and tanks.

We responded with fast and accurate gunfire. It was during this period of the patrol when a bullet struck the turret and shrapnel from the bullet hit my helmet, launching me backwards into the rear of the vehicle. I was dazed and shocked but got back to my feet quickly and observed for any other threats.

Once the incident was over, we moved position again to continue the patrol. Immediately there was the sound of a bang and a loud explosion close by. We were informed that the terrorist leader had been killed. We drove to our hold position before heading back to base. We parked at the roadside in the centre of Basra, opposite the terrorist car. Black smoke billowed from the car which was still on fire and there was a strong smell of burning flesh. Observing the burning bodies in the vehicle shocked me to the core. We headed back to base with everyone concerned about our fallen comrades. I was in a state of shock and sat quietly until we finished the patrol.

The remainder of the tour continued with constant incidents of gunfire while on patrol and sleepless days due to indirect mortar fire, but it was the loss of life that significantly affected us all. The toil of the operational tour started to profoundly affect the morale of the regiment and the desire to go home played on everyone's minds.

The timings for leaving were staggered, due to flights and the process of going through decompression training in Cyprus. The decompression training was to allow soldiers to re-enter society and non-conflict environment without the pressure of interactions. However, it was not easy to transition from the traumatic exposures of the combat actions that I had experienced during the Iraq tour to then relax and decompress while participating in in-group sporting activities. I usually enjoyed playing sports. However, I found it difficult to concentrate and enjoy them with my mind still pondering my time in Iraq. The nighttime was social time with everyone being encouraged to participate in drinking alcohol.

I found the decompression-training period of two days in Cyprus being in the company of soldiers I had served in Iraq with a very negative experience. It was a very forced environment and offered no consideration to how I or anyone else may be feeling from our experiences in Iraq. I was expected to perform normally, while the traumatic experiences from the tour weighed heavy on my mind and impacted on my mental health. The Iraq tour had been extremely challenging, but the decompression training provided no counselling support.

The flight back to the UK was a big event, with plans for family and friends to welcome us back at camp. However, I did not want a big fanfare and was in no rush to see anyone on my return. As we drove into camp, families stood with flags and banners with everyone cheering us home with the band playing music, but I needed to escape. There did not seem much to celebrate.

I quickly handed in my rifle and promptly did my tasks before I was allowed to begin post-deployment leave, but instead of rushing off to enjoy civilian life, I hid away in my room for three days. The decision to self-isolate helped me to not upset family and friends with talking about what Iraq was really like. Still, hiding away from everyone caused me to avoid the traumatic issues that caused me distress. I knew something was wrong, but I could not understand it or find a way forward or seek help.

Battle with Post-Traumatic Stress Disorder

The next phase of my Army career allowed me to use my experience and knowledge as an instructor at both Winchester and Pirbright training camps. The opportunity to train recruits filled me with pride and desire to give them the best support possible to transition becoming a soldier. I remembered how hard basic training was for me and having positive role models helped me complete basic training.

I decided to work hard in making the experience an enjoyable one with challenging real-life scenarios to help nurture and develop the recruits under my command. I was in Winchester, which had me working with junior soldiers, similar to the age that I enlisted in 1989. I was instructed by my commanders that the age of the new recruits determined the methods, pace, and tone that I delivered the subject matter during basic training. However, when I moved to Pirbright, the demographic of the new recruits was between 18 and 32 years of age. Basic training for adult recruits was only 14 weeks, which altered the method delivery due to the pressure of the timetable and allowed a more robust instructional approach.

Teaching at the training establishment maintained a fast-paced working environment; as soon as one platoon finished, and another would start. Being busy suited me because during the summer when I had no recruits, demons would haunt me. My colleagues commented that I elicited angry and aggressive behaviours and shouted during conversations. I struggled with sleep, due to my mind being full of memories of my tour of Iraq and I relived traumatic events.

My response was to ignore the memories, work harder, and push myself at fitness so that I would feel exhausted; all in effort to ward off the demons. It did not work. When I had lots of time on my hands, I found myself drinking to help me sleep and to stop the dark memories affecting my every thought.

The dark days took over and the traumatic memories began a period which saw me spiral out of control. Heavy drinking significantly compromised my decision-making processes. I was afraid to stop drinking but equally ignorant of what impact my behaviour had on others. I could not permit myself to be seen as weak so instead of seeking help I hid it from everyone.

My heavy drinking had finally caught up with me when I was stopped for drink driving. The military had rules and standards against drink driving. Following my arrest, I had effectively damaged my credibility and jeopardised any chance of my Army career continuing on the same path.

My career almost certain to be over, I began to accept the need for medical support; and while I knew I was struggling genuinely on the inside, it took this shameful act to make people aware that I was in pain. I went to see my doctor, who quickly recognised symptoms similar to PTSD; he prescribed medication and arranged a psychological assessment.

While awaiting punishment for drink driving, I had weekly counselling sessions that were helping me to understand what was causing my distress. I was seen as the black sheep around camp with my commanders alienating me from my support network. Instead of providing a duty of care, they told me to get my "head out of the sand" and "man up". They ignored my medical condition.

Finally, I was charged with drink driving and part of the disciplinary procedure would remove me from my role as an instructor in Pirbright and return me to my regiment in Catterick Garrison. I would be provided with no medical support for over three months due to the delay in transferring my treatment records.

In December 2013, the head of the psychology department at the Duchess of Kent Military Hospital (DKMH) finally saw me. During my initial assessment, I had a very emotional and detailed discussion in which I had remarked on the very traumatic events that I had experienced during my Iraq tour. It was following this initial assessment that I was diagnosed with PTSD. It was recommended that I should be medically discharged due to the impact of PTSD and remaining in a military environment was having on me. I left my regiment the next day and finished the remainder of my career with the support of the "help for heroes" staff at Phoenix House, who helped me with the transition from military to civilian life.

I served over 25 years in the Army, representing my regiment in multiple operational environments, which went on to affect the quality of my life. My chain of command ignored me or punished me when I needed their support, especially when I did not understand why my troubles were escalating out of control.

I completed my Army career and should feel proud of this achievement. Still, due to the harsh treatment I received from my superiors and the impact PTSD has had on my mental health and well-being, this has left me ashamed of my career. While I continue my fight with PTSD, I question my life and worry about what my future holds. I am not the only soldier to worry.

The Growing Concern of Post-Traumatic Stress Disorder in the British Military

Following the end of military conflict in the Gulf, The United Kingdom's military personnel returned home, with many exhibiting the psychological impact of being exposed to life-threatening events (Grillon, & Morgan III, 1999; Spoont et al., 2010). The exposure to military combat, human-caused disasters, and loss of life leaves many soldiers displaying symptoms linked to Post-Traumatic Stress Disorder (PTSD) (Van der Kolk, & Najavits, 2013).

Post-Traumatic Stress Disorder (PTSD) is a complex life-debilitating anxiety disorder that can develop when exposed to life-threatening, traumatic, or extremely distressing events (Hamblen, 2009; Thomas et al., 2010). It is a prominent mental health issue within both the military and veteran communities (Van der Kolk & Najavits 2013). Since 2016, there has been a documented 17% increase of UK veterans being affected compared with 4.5% of the UK adult population (Leightley et al., 2019).

PTSD consists of four symptom clusters which include the re-experiencing of extremely traumatic events through nightmares and disturbing memories, mood behaviour changes, hyperarousal, and the avoidance of reminders of traumatic events (Monson, Taft, & Fredman, 2009). Subsequently, PTSD can have a multifaceted impact on veterans, with individuals expressing noticeable changes such as the loss of productivity, impaired cognitive performance, alterations in brain function, as well as documented cases of chronic diseases (Mobbs, & Bonanno, 2018; Solomon et al., 2012).

PTSD symptoms deeply affect veterans' quality of life, especially the manifestation of re-experiencing a traumatic event. Studies have found that veterans who have PTSD have also presented higher rates of metabolic disorder, diabetes, and obesity (Bartoli et al., 2015; Buta et al., 2018). Furthermore, veterans with PTSD often exhibited decreased levels of participation in regular physical exercise which has likely contributed to a worrying increase in cognitive and medical comorbidities heavily related to a sedentary lifestyle (Celano et al., 2016; Greenbaum et al., 2017).

The current pharmacological and psychological treatments are proven to be effective treatment methods when dealing with some characteristic symptoms of PTSD. However, many veterans are left untreated or supported due to barriers of PTSD, which include stigma, self-efficacy, and access to appropriate medical care (Fitelson et al., 2011; Forbes et al., 2008 2008). The traditional mental health treatments for PTSD often consist of cognitive therapies, psychiatric-led sessions and general health issues associated with PTSD (Ehlers et al., 2005; Karlin et al., 2010).

It is essential to consider the efficacy of all treatment pathways before prescribing treatment to veterans who have PTSD, including holistic and physical exercise as a practical alternative to treatment (Oppizzi, & Umberger, 2018; Possemato et al., 2011).

Research highlights that physical exercise is a viable therapeutic modality for mental health issues, including depression and PTSD (De Vries et al., 2012; Rosenbaum et al., 2015). Physical exercise is an activity that requires physical effort, and when carried out safely, will also sustain or improve health and fitness (De Vries et al., 2012; Gates et al., 2012) to help ward off other health issues resulting from a secondary lifestyle. Physical exercise thus has been prescribed as a method of rehabilitation from injury, as well as aiding the improvement of mental well-being (Bartels et al., 2014).

I do not claim to offer clinical diagnoses or medical solutions. Instead, I write as a veteran, a scholar, and someone living with PTSD who has found meaning and partial relief through physical activity. My goal is not only to share my story but to contribute to a deeper, more nuanced understanding of trauma and recovery, one that recognises the body, identity, and masculine culture as central to the healing process.

This chapter has presented a candid and emotionally grounded account of my lived experience with PTSD following military service. Through reflective narrative, I have explored how trauma reshaped my sense of self, influenced by the silence and stoicism embedded in military masculinity. In grounding this monograph in personal experience, I hope to offer not just data or theory, but a human context that challenges conventional clinical perspectives and invites new conversations about embodied healing, identity, and post-traumatic growth.

References

Bartels, S. J., Pratt, S. I., Mueser, K. T., Forester, B. P., Wolfe, R., Cather, C., ... & Feldman, J. (2014). Long-term outcomes of a randomized trial of integrated skills training and preventive healthcare for older adults with serious mental illness. *The American Journal of Geriatric Psychiatry, 22*(11), 1251–1261.

Bartoli, F., Crocamo, C., Alamia, A., et al. (2015). Posttraumatic stress disorder and risk of obesity: Systematic review and meta-analysis. *Journal of Clinical Psychiatry, 76*(10), 1253–1261.

Buta, B., Maselko, J., & Kramer, J. (2018). PTSD and metabolic syndrome in veterans. *Annals of Epidemiology, 28*(1), 1–7.

Celano, C. M., Daunis, D. J., Lokko, H. N., Campbell, K. A., & Huffman, J. C. (2016). Anxiety disorders and cardiovascular disease. *Current Psychiatry Reports, 18*(11), Article 101.

De Vries, J. D., van Hooff, M. L., Geurts, S. A., & Kompier, M. A. (2012). Exercise as an intervention to reduce stress. *Journal of Occupational Health Psychology, 17*(3), 210–219.

Ehlers, A., Clark, D. M. Hackmann, A., McManus, F., & Fennell, M., (2005). Cognitive therapy for PTSD: Development and evaluation. *Behaviour Research and Therapy, 43*(4), 413–431.

Fitelson, E., Kim, S., Baker, A. S., & Leight, K. (2011). Treatment of postpartum depression: Clinical, psychological and social perspectives. *International Journal of Women's Health, 3*, 1–14.

Forbes, D., Parslow, R., Creamer, M., Allen, N., McHugh, T., & Hopwood, M. (2008). Mechanisms of anger and treatment outcome in combat veterans with posttraumatic stress disorder. *Journal of Traumatic Stress: Official Publication of The International Society for Traumatic Stress Studies, 21*(2), 142–149.

Gates, N., Singh, M. A. F., Sachdev, P. S., & Valenzuela, M. J. (2012). Cognitive and physical exercise as intervention for age-related cognitive decline. *Clinical Interventions in Aging, 7*, 45–57.

Greenbaum, M. A., Neylan, T. C., & Rosen, C. S. (2017). Exercise as a treatment for PTSD. *Current Psychiatry Reports, 19*(8), Article 57.

Grillon, C., & Morgan, C. A., III. (1999). Fear-potentiated startle in the human nervous system. *Biological Psychiatry, 46*(10), 1455–1463.

Hamblen, J. L. (2009). PTSD overview. National Centre for PTSD (Fact Sheet).

Karlin, B. E., Ruzek, J. I., Eftekhari, A., Monson, C. M., Hembree, E. A., ... & Foa, E. B.Chard, K. M., et al. (2010). Dissemination of evidence-based treatments for PTSD in the Veterans Health Administration. *Journal of Traumatic Stress, 23*(6), 663–673.

Leightley, D., Puddephatt, Leightley, D., Palmer, L., Jones, N., Mahmoodi, T., Drummond, C., ... & Goodwin, L. (2019). A qualitative evaluation of the acceptability of a tailored smartphone alcohol intervention for a military population: information about drinking for ex-serving personnel (InDEx) app. *JMIR mHealth and uHealth, 7*(5), e12267.

Mobbs, D., & Bonanno, G. A. (2018). Brain mechanisms for resilience and PTSD. *Nature Neuroscience, 21*(2), 158–166.

Monson, C. M., Taft, C. T., & Fredman, S. J. (2009). Military-related PTSD and intimate relationships. *Behaviour Therapy, 40*(3), 276–291.

Oppizzi, L. M., & Umberger, R. (2018). The use of exercise to manage PTSD symptoms. *Military Medicine, 183*(5–6), e219–e226.

Possemato, K., Wade, M., Andersen, J., & Ouimette, P. (2011). Exercise in the treatment of PTSD. *Psychiatric Annals, 41*(9), 546–552.

Rosenbaum, S., Vancampfort, D., Steel, Z., Newby, J., Ward, P. B., & Stubbs, B. (2015). Physical activity and PTSD: A systematic review and meta-analysis. *Psychiatry Research, 230*(2), 130–136.

Solomon, Z., Mikulincer, M., & Shaver, P. R. (2012). PTSD and physical illness: Mechanisms and manifestations. *Psychological Trauma: Theory, Research, Practice, and Policy, 4*(1), 46–53.

Spoont, M. R., Murdoch, M., Hodges, J., & Nugent, S. (2010). Barriers to care in veterans with PTSD. *Journal of Traumatic Stress, 23*(5), 654–662.

Thomas, J. L., Wilk, J. E., Riviere, L. A., McGurk, D., Castro, C. A., & Hoge, C. W. (2010). et al. (2010). Prevalence of mental health problems in Iraq and Afghanistan veterans. *Journal of Traumatic Stress, 23*(1), 20–27.

Van der Kolk, B. A., & Najavits, L. M. (2013). PTSD, substance use and comorbidity. *American Journal of Psychiatry, 170*(1), 19–21.

CHAPTER 2

PTSD in Military Men: Masculinities, Symptomology, and Treatment

Understanding post-traumatic stress disorder (PTSD) in military populations requires an analysis that goes beyond diagnostic categories to explore the social and cultural forces that shape its development, presentation, and treatment. Central among these forces is masculinity, particularly the hegemonic forms that dominate military life. Traditional military masculinities valorise emotional control, physical endurance, stoicism, and self-reliance. These attributes, while advantageous in combat, often become psychological liabilities in post-service life. They can prevent men from recognising symptoms of trauma, inhibit help-seeking, and complicate therapeutic engagement. This chapter critically examines the genesis of PTSD in military history, the symptomology that defines it in clinical contexts, and the current treatment modalities available. In each section, we interrogate how masculinities influence veterans' experiences, shaping their perceptions of distress, their willingness to access care, and the clinical strategies best suited to support their recovery.

Masculinities and Mental Health: PTSD Genesis

The history of post-traumatic stress disorder (PTSD) is deeply intertwined with the evolution of psychiatric knowledge and societal constructions of masculinity. While PTSD only gained official status in the DSM-III in 1980 (Connell, 2016), psychological responses to trauma have been

J. Alder, *Military Men, Physical Exercise, and Post-Traumatic Stress Disorder*, Palgrave Studies in Masculinity, Sport and Exercise,
https://doi.org/10.1007/978-3-032-08957-1_2

recorded throughout military history. Terms such as "Nostalgia", "Irritable Heart", and "Soldier's Heart" reveal how emotional suffering was historically repackaged into socially acceptable diagnoses that aligned with dominant gender norms. In militarised settings, masculinity has traditionally been equated with stoicism, control, and resilience. Consequently, the open expression of distress was pathologised or interpreted as weakness. These gendered expectations have long shaped not only how psychological symptoms were diagnosed and treated, but also how soldiers experienced and understood their own mental health (Batcho, 2013; Sharif et al., 2018).

Military masculinity has often demanded that men suppress fear and emotion, even in the face of horror. During the American Civil War, diagnoses such as "Irritable Heart" allowed clinicians to explain symptoms of anxiety and emotional exhaustion without challenging masculine ideals (Smith et al., 2014). These soldiers were typically treated with rest and reassignment, not therapy, reflecting an institutional focus on maintaining operational efficiency rather than addressing psychological suffering. This model of treatment reinforced the notion that combat trauma could and should be overcome without emotional breakdown, reinforcing stigma against those who could not conform.

The First World War marked a significant transformation in the visibility of combat trauma with the emergence of the term "Shell Shock". The scale and brutality of trench warfare exposed many soldiers to relentless psychological stress. Symptoms including tremors, mutism, and dissociation were observed in large numbers, yet medical and military authorities were often reluctant to acknowledge their origins in emotional trauma. Many soldiers diagnosed with Shell Shock were subjected to harsh discipline, reflecting the belief that their condition stemmed from moral or personal failure (Loughran, 2012; Alker & Godfrey, 2016). This perception was deeply rooted in the prevailing ideology of hegemonic masculinity, which viewed emotional vulnerability as antithetical to the soldier's role.

The treatment of Shell Shock was shaped by the principles of "Forward Psychiatry" or "PIE"—proximity, immediacy, and expectation of recovery (Jones & Wessely, 2003). These principles aimed to return men to the front line rather than provide meaningful psychological intervention. While the approach reduced long-term hospitalisations, it reinforced the imperative to "perform" masculinity by quickly overcoming trauma. The goal was not holistic recovery but rather the restoration of military function, demonstrating how psychiatric practices aligned with cultural expectations of male endurance.

Freud's psychoanalytic model of "War Neurosis" provided an alternative explanation for trauma, framing it as a psychic conflict between a soldier's pre-war ego and the new identity formed under extreme stress (Danto, 2016, Freud, 2016). Although Freud's ideas introduced the possibility of unconscious processes contributing to psychological breakdown, they continued to reflect gendered assumptions. Emotional expression in men was often seen as regression, while hysteria was commonly feminised in clinical literature (Leeb, 2018). Freud's theories thus operated within a framework that implicitly reinforced binary notions of strength and weakness, further entrenching the marginalisation of traumatised men.

The Second World War saw the introduction of new diagnostic terms, such as "Combat Fatigue" and "Battle Exhaustion", which were intended to be less stigmatising than Shell Shock (Bliese et al., 2011). Nevertheless, the underlying assumptions about masculinity remained largely unchanged. Psychological casualties were still viewed as liabilities, and the expectation was that men would recover quickly and return to duty. Medical interventions, including sedation, brief counselling, and reconditioning, were applied with the same goal: to restore the soldier's capacity to function under pressure.

American psychiatrist Abram Kardiner challenged the idea that combat trauma was fundamentally different from civilian trauma. He argued that the neuroses experienced by soldiers were similar to those seen in victims of accidents and assaults, thereby universalising the concept of trauma (Levandoski, 2010). However, Kardiner's perspective was not widely accepted at the time, and institutional resistance to emotional vulnerability in men persisted. Military and psychiatric systems continued to reflect and reinforce cultural expectations that equated masculinity with emotional control.

The Vietnam War exposed the limitations of these approaches. Soldiers returning from Vietnam displayed symptoms now recognisable as PTSD: intrusive memories, emotional detachment, irritability, and hypervigilance. However, many faced societal rejection and institutional neglect. The term "Post-Vietnam Syndrome" emerged to describe these symptoms, but formal recognition was delayed due to the ongoing reluctance to legitimise psychological suffering in male veterans. The broader social context of civil unrest, anti-war activism, and changes in public attitudes created space for a more open discussion of trauma, culminating in the inclusion of PTSD in the DSM-III.

While the DSM-III's recognition of PTSD in 1980 represented a clinical milestone, the diagnosis remained shaped by gendered assumptions. The conceptualisation of PTSD was based on a model of acute trauma followed by measurable symptoms. However, this framework did not adequately address the chronic, socially mediated nature of trauma for many veterans. Moreover, masculinity continued to act as a barrier to treatment. Many men resisted diagnosis, fearing that it would mark them as weak, unstable, or unmanly (Owens et al., 2012). Research indicates that male veterans often avoid mental health services or delay seeking help until symptoms become unmanageable (Kinghorn, 2015).

In the post-9/11 era, the wars in Iraq and Afghanistan brought renewed focus to PTSD, particularly in relation to comorbid conditions such as Traumatic Brain Injury (TBI). Advances in protective gear and medical evacuation allowed more soldiers to survive, but many returned with complex psychological and cognitive injuries (Mulherkar & Tolias, 2020). Symptoms such as memory loss, irritability, and emotional dysregulation blur the lines between PTSD and TBI, complicating diagnosis and treatment. Research also suggests that some veterans may prefer a diagnosis of TBI because it aligns with the cultural acceptability of physical injury, avoiding the stigma associated with mental illness (Elbogen et al., 2019).

Studies have also investigated the possible link between PTSD and Chronic Traumatic Encephalopathy (CTE), a neurodegenerative disease associated with repeated head trauma. Veterans exposed to multiple blast events and concussive forces often display symptoms similar to those observed in athletes with CTE (French et al., 2020). The pathophysiological overlap between PTSD, TBI, and CTE challenges traditional diagnostic boundaries and raises questions about how trauma is embodied and gendered. Physical explanations for psychological symptoms may be more palatable within a masculine framework, but they risk obscuring the emotional dimensions of trauma that require psychological intervention.

Gender-sensitive approaches to trauma have gained traction in recent years, emphasising the importance of addressing masculinity directly within therapeutic contexts. Interventions that incorporate discussions about military culture and masculine identity can reduce stigma and improve outcomes. Psychoeducation Programmes that normalise emotional expression and reframe help-seeking as an act of strength rather than weakness have shown promise. Group therapy models that foster solidarity among veterans can also help to reconfigure harmful gender norms and create a safe space for emotional exploration.

Therapists and clinicians must also be aware of the role that masculine identity plays in shaping both symptom expression and recovery trajectories. For many veterans, military service is not just an occupation but a foundational aspect of selfhood. Psychological injury can thus be experienced as a profound rupture in identity. Treatment must engage with this existential dimension, helping veterans navigate the loss of the soldier self and build new narratives of masculinity that allow for vulnerability, reflection, and emotional connection.

While the inclusion of PTSD in diagnostic frameworks such as the DSM and ICD has improved access to care, it has not eliminated the cultural stigma surrounding emotional suffering in men. Masculinity continues to function as both a risk factor for trauma and a barrier to recovery. Hegemonic masculine norms discourage help-seeking, limit emotional vocabulary, and promote isolation, all of which contribute to the chronicity of PTSD in male veterans (Connell & Messerschmidt, 2005; Ross et al., 2018).

As the field of trauma studies continues to evolve, it is essential to centre gender in both research and clinical practice. Masculinity must be understood not as a static identity but as a dynamic social construct that influences how trauma is experienced, interpreted, and addressed. Psychiatric frameworks must move beyond symptom checklists to incorporate a more holistic understanding of trauma that recognises the intersections of gender, identity, and social context.

Future models of care must be inclusive and intersectional, recognising that not all men experience masculinity in the same way. Factors such as race, class, sexuality, and military rank also shape how PTSD is understood and treated. A more nuanced understanding of masculinities can help clinicians tailor interventions to meet the diverse needs of male veterans and reduce disparities in treatment outcomes.

The relationship between PTSD and masculinity is neither incidental nor superficial. It is foundational to the historical, clinical, and cultural construction of trauma. Understanding this relationship is essential not only for improving therapeutic outcomes but also for challenging the broader systems that perpetuate silence, shame, and suffering among those most affected by war.

PTSD Causes, Comorbidities, and Symptomologies in Military Veterans: A Focus on Masculinities

Post-Traumatic Stress Disorder (PTSD) remains one of the most complex and debilitating psychological conditions afflicting military veterans, particularly those exposed to the cumulative traumas of combat. Battlefield experiences, including persistent life threats, moral injuries, and exposure to death, are principal precipitators of PTSD. These events often leave veterans grappling with long-term impairments in emotional regulation, cognitive processing, and physical well-being. Military service frequently places individuals in hyper-intense environments where threat is pervasive and chronic, with limited opportunity for decompression or emotional processing. The prolonged exposure to trauma contributes to enduring psychological sequelae (Abeyasinghe et al., 2012; Yehuda et al., 2014).

The Diagnostic and Statistical Manual of Mental Disorders (DSM-V) outlines four core symptom clusters that characterise PTSD: (1) intrusive re-experiencing of traumatic events, (2) active avoidance of trauma-related stimuli, (3) pervasive negative alterations in cognition and mood, and (4) heightened physiological arousal and reactivity. These clusters provide a structured understanding of the disorder, yet military-specific trauma responses often transcend textbook classifications. Among Iraq and Afghanistan veterans, for instance, studies indicate that roughly one in five meet the diagnostic threshold for PTSD. These figures may underrepresent actual prevalence due to underreporting, which is often fuelled by institutional stigma and internalised masculine ideals.

Intrusive symptoms often manifest through distressing recollections, recurrent nightmares, and vivid flashbacks. These cognitive intrusions not only impair sleep quality and daily functioning but also reinforce a persistent sense of threat, keeping veterans psychologically tethered to past traumas (Andrewes & Jenkins, 2019; Murphy et al., 2016). Neuroimaging studies have revealed hyperactivity in the amygdala, coupled with impaired regulation by the medial prefrontal cortex and hippocampus, neural pathways associated with fear, memory, and emotional modulation (Akiki et al., 2017). The result is a loop of heightened arousal and impaired emotional regulation. For male veterans especially, this internal chaos is often concealed beneath an exterior of control and strength, aligning with sociocultural expectations of masculinity. Yet such concealment can intensify distress, increase isolation, and disrupt relationships.

Avoidance, the second cluster, often includes both behavioural and cognitive strategies to elude trauma reminders. Veterans may disengage from relationships, avoid public spaces, or repress distressing memories. These actions are not simply self-protective; they are also shaped by masculine ideals that equate vulnerability with weakness (Church, 2010). Consequently, substance misuse, particularly alcohol, is frequently employed as a form of emotional numbing. Some veterans report drinking excessively to cope with hypervigilance or to induce sleep. Even while deployed, service members report relying on rigid routines, intense physical training, or books and films to distract from stressors. However, these temporary fixes often fail to address the underlying psychological injury.

Negative alterations in cognition and mood, such as chronic guilt, shame, and detachment, often represent a deep internalisation of trauma. These symptoms not only erode the veteran's sense of self but also inhibit their capacity for intimacy, empathy, and positive self-regard. Moral injury, resulting from perceived transgressions of deeply held beliefs such as killing in combat or surviving when comrades did not, frequently underpins such symptoms. Shame and guilt may be intensified by masculine codes of honour, which valorise strength, protection, and control (Brock & Lettini, 2012). The perceived failure to uphold these standards in the face of trauma can precipitate depressive symptoms, hopelessness, and suicidal ideation.

This cluster intersects with broader discourses of masculinity. The military fosters a culture steeped in traditional masculine norms including emotional stoicism, endurance, physical power, and hierarchical dominance. Emotional suppression, often encouraged in training and deployment, becomes internalised and habitual, impeding help-seeking post-deployment. For male veterans, expressing emotional vulnerability is often perceived as incompatible with the warrior identity. As Shields et al. argue, distress is frequently construed as weakness, reinforcing silence and diminishing therapeutic engagement. This cultural coding of masculinity obstructs recovery, delays clinical intervention, and exacerbates symptoms. The internal conflict between lived psychological distress and the pressure to maintain masculine ideals undermines self-compassion, perpetuates emotional detachment, and alienates the individual from potential sources of support.

Hyperarousal, manifested in exaggerated startle responses, irritability, and hypervigilance, further challenges post-military reintegration. This cluster reflects a physiological state of continued alertness, shaped by dysregulation of the hypothalamic-pituitary-adrenal (HPA) axis and overactivation of sympathetic nervous system responses (Van der Kolk, 1994). Elevated cortisol and norepinephrine levels prolong physiological stress responses, contributing to cardiovascular, metabolic, and immune system dysregulation. This state is not only exhausting but also isolating. Veterans often struggle to relax in civilian environments. In male-dominated spaces, however, irritability and anger may be normalised or even valorised, enabling the performance of strength and dominance at the expense of psychological stability. Consequently, expressions of anger may function as both coping strategies and as affirmations of masculine identity, reinforcing a damaging cycle that inhibits emotional processing.

PTSD is rarely experienced in isolation. Comorbidities such as substance abuse, major depressive disorder, generalised anxiety, and self-harming behaviours are commonly reported among veterans. Substance misuse, particularly alcohol and prescription medication, is frequently used to manage intrusive symptoms or emotional numbing. Additionally, veterans may experience eating disorders, suicidal ideation, and personality disturbances. The result is a complex clinical picture that requires integrated treatment models to address both trauma and co-occurring disorders. Poor sleep, impaired concentration, and strained relationships further degrade quality of life. These secondary effects may be interpreted as personal failures within masculinised frameworks, further entrenching self-blame and delaying treatment.

Understanding comorbidities through a gendered lens reveals additional complexities. Within hegemonic masculinity, emotional self-disclosure is discouraged, leading veterans to mask psychological pain through behaviours that appear socially acceptable within male peer groups. Drinking, aggression, and risk-taking are not only symptomatic but also performative, allowing men to avoid confronting psychological distress while still conforming to masculine codes. This pattern of maladaptive coping is particularly pronounced among younger veterans who may lack robust social or therapeutic support networks. Mental health services must therefore actively challenge gender norms that inhibit self-care and reframe help-seeking as an act of strength rather than weakness.

Physical comorbidities also demand attention. Many veterans with PTSD experience chronic pain, metabolic dysfunction, and cardiovascular issues. These may stem from the physiological toll of sustained hyper-arousal, medication side effects, or lifestyle factors such as poor sleep and diet (Bartoli et al., 2015). Veterans often seek medical support for these issues before disclosing psychological symptoms, highlighting the need for trauma-informed practice across primary care settings. Treating PTSD thus requires an interdisciplinary approach that integrates medical, psychological, and social dimensions of care.

Another complicating factor is the co-occurrence of PTSD with traumatic brain injury (TBI), a condition frequently sustained during military service. TBI and PTSD often present overlapping symptoms, including irritability, emotional dysregulation, and memory problems. The dual burden of physical and psychological trauma complicates diagnosis and requires tailored interventions that consider the interaction of neurobiological and emotional impairments. Misattribution of symptoms to one condition may result in inadequate treatment and reinforce cycles of frustration and disengagement.

In summary, PTSD in military veterans is a multifaceted condition that must be understood within biopsychosocial and gendered frameworks. The DSM-V provides a useful clinical taxonomy, but a fuller understanding emerges when symptom clusters are situated within the lived realities of military masculinities, trauma histories, and comorbid conditions. Veterans' psychological distress is not only shaped by individual pathology but also by institutional cultures that valorise emotional control, physical resilience, and stoicism. Such norms obstruct recovery, alienate individuals from supportive networks, and contribute to high rates of treatment dropout. Effective interventions must challenge these masculinised narratives and normalise emotional expression and vulnerability as part of the recovery journey. Only then can treatment begin to align with the real-world needs of those who have served.

Current Treatment Modalities for PTSD and the Role of Masculinities

Post-traumatic stress disorder (PTSD) remains one of the most prevalent and complex psychological disorders affecting military veterans. Since its formal recognition in the third edition of the Diagnostic and Statistical Manual of Mental Disorders (DSM-III) in 1980, treatment modalities have significantly evolved. Initial interventions primarily focused on restoring general psychological stability without directly targeting the trauma-related symptoms that characterise PTSD. As diagnostic criteria and clinical understanding advanced, so too did the specificity and efficacy of interventions. Yet despite this progress, many veterans, particularly male veterans, remain hesitant to access care. This reluctance is not only a result of stigma and institutional mistrust but is deeply entwined with internalised masculine norms of stoicism, autonomy, and emotional restraint (Fitelson et al., 2011; Forbes et al., 2012).

Modern PTSD treatments are typically divided into three categories: psychological, pharmacological, and emerging or holistic interventions. These are delivered within two key phases: first-line treatments, which have robust empirical support and are usually initiated early in care, and second-line treatments, which are offered when first-line interventions are ineffective or contraindicated. These categories are further complicated by veterans' personal experiences, symptom profiles, and beliefs about mental health care, many of which are shaped by military training and masculine identity.

Table 2.1 summarises the foundational psychological therapies used for PTSD. Among psychological therapies, Cognitive Behavioural Therapy (CBT) is considered the foundational first-line treatment. CBT involves structured, time-limited techniques aimed at altering distorted beliefs, processing traumatic memories, and improving emotional regulation (Monson et al., 2006; Karlin et al., 2010). Cognitive Processing Therapy (CPT), a subtype of CBT, focuses on modifying maladaptive trauma-related thoughts, while Prolonged Exposure Therapy systematically desensitises individuals to traumatic cues by encouraging controlled re-experiencing of trauma memories. These therapies have high success rates, but for many male veterans, participation is undermined by traditional masculine ideals that discourage emotional disclosure. These veterans may struggle to articulate internal distress or perceive therapy as a challenge to their autonomy and strength (Wampold et al., 2010).

Eye Movement Desensitisation and Reprocessing (EMDR) is another prominent intervention, typically employed as a second-line therapy. EMDR involves the guided reprocessing of trauma through bilateral sensory stimulation, such as eye movements, to reduce emotional reactivity (Maxfield & Hyer, 2002). Though evidence supports EMDR's efficacy, especially in civilian populations, it can be perceived as intrusive or incompatible with masculine performance scripts. Veterans often express discomfort with emotionally immersive treatments, particularly those that do

Table 2.1 First-line and second-line treatments for PTSD

PTSD treatments	*First line*	*Second line*
Psychological	Cognitive Behavioural Therapy (CBT) Cognitive Processing Therapy (CPT) Prolonged Exposure Therapy	Eye Movement Desensitisation and Reprocessing (EMDR)
Pharmacological	Antidepressants (e.g., Sertraline, Paroxetine, Fluoxetine, Venlafaxine)	Nefazodone Mirtazapine Tricyclic Antidepressants Monoamine Oxidase Inhibitors (MAOIs) Prazosin

Note: This classification reflects clinical guidelines for the treatment of PTSD and highlights both established and adjunctive interventions

This table summarises commonly prescribed psychological and pharmacological treatments, organised by clinical recommendation phase

not align with their perceptions of control or composure (Davidson & Parker, 2001; Valiente-Gómez et al., 2017; Hurley, 2018).

Pharmacological approaches are often used concurrently with or following psychological interventions. First-line medications typically include selective serotonin reuptake inhibitors (SSRIs), such as sertraline, paroxetine, fluoxetine, and venlafaxine. These medications work by modulating neurotransmitter levels to reduce symptoms of anxiety, intrusive memories, and low mood. However, pharmacotherapy may be seen by some veterans as a concession to weakness or as a loss of autonomy, particularly among those who embrace self-reliant masculine identities (MacManus et al., 2012; Singh et al., 2018). Moreover, the side effects of SSRIs, including emotional numbing and sexual dysfunction, may further alienate patients from their sense of identity and agency (Brewin, Garnett & Andrews, 2011).

When SSRIs prove ineffective or are poorly tolerated, second-line pharmacological treatments are introduced. These include mirtazapine for insomnia and depressive symptoms, tricyclic antidepressants, monoamine oxidase inhibitors (MAOIs), and Prazosin, which is specifically used to reduce nightmares and hyperarousal (Raskind et al., 2013). Nefazodone has also been explored in cases where other antidepressants are not well suited. While these treatments can be effective, they often require long-term compliance and close monitoring. Veterans who equate medication with dependency or a failure of will, may disengage, undermining therapeutic outcomes.

As traditional models show limited success in some veteran populations, there is increasing interest in alternative, holistic, and non-conventional approaches. These include yoga, mindfulness-based stress reduction, acupuncture, and even psychedelic-assisted therapy, such as 3,4-methylenedioxymethamphetamine (MDMA). Holistic modalities appeal to many veterans because they incorporate embodied practices and physical movement, which feel more congruent with masculine-coded traits such as strength, discipline, and control. Yoga and meditation, in particular, have been found to regulate heart rate variability, decrease cortisol levels, and reduce anxiety symptoms (Williston et al., 2020).

MDMA-assisted therapy is currently in the final stages of clinical trials and has shown significant promise in enabling emotional openness and deeper trauma processing. MDMA reduces fear responses and increases empathic engagement, allowing veterans to access and process painful memories that are otherwise suppressed (Mitchell et al., 2021; Varker et al., 2021). However, some veterans remain wary of such therapies due to perceived risks, cultural associations with drug misuse, and internalised codes of discipline and emotional control (Passie, 2018).

Masculine identity continues to shape how veterans approach and interpret treatment. Many male veterans minimise symptoms, deny distress, or present with emotional detachment to maintain control or avoid perceived emasculation. These behaviours are deeply rooted in military culture, where self-sufficiency, resilience, and mission-focus are central tenets (MacManus et al., 2012). Consequently, traditional therapeutic environments may feel foreign or uncomfortable. Without a trauma-informed, gender-sensitive approach, clinicians risk losing rapport, under-diagnosing symptoms, and increasing dropout rates.

Practitioners who integrate gender-awareness into treatment planning, by acknowledging the friction between emotional openness and masculine norms, are more likely to retain veterans in therapy. This can include offering male-only groups, integrating physical activity into care plans, or using language that aligns with veterans' values of strength and control. CrossFit, martial arts, and team sports like rugby can serve as gateways into healing by promoting structure, camaraderie, and physical mastery. These activities create emotionally safe environments where psychological recovery can occur without overtly challenging masculine identities (Oppizzi & Umberger, 2018).

In summary, effective PTSD treatment requires more than a knowledge of symptomology or pharmacology. It requires a comprehensive understanding of the sociocultural landscape that shapes help-seeking behaviour and therapeutic engagement. For military veterans, particularly men, trauma recovery is influenced not just by what therapies are available, but by how those therapies intersect with their sense of identity, masculinity, and meaning. Integrating this awareness into clinical care is essential for improving outcomes and developing interventions that are not only evidence-based, but also context-sensitive and culturally competent.

Chapter Conclusion

PTSD in military veterans cannot be understood, or effectively treated, without considering the pervasive influence of masculinity. From its historical conceptualisation as "Shell Shock" to its formal recognition in modern diagnostic manuals, PTSD has been interpreted and managed within gendered frameworks that prioritise endurance over vulnerability. The symptomology of PTSD often clashes with military norms of self-control, leading many men to suppress emotional distress or reinterpret it through physical or behavioural symptoms. These patterns frequently result in delayed diagnosis and reduced engagement with psychological care. Even within current treatment modalities, whether psychological, pharmacological, or alternative, the tension between masculine identity and emotional openness remains a central challenge. However, emerging gender-sensitive approaches offer hope. By acknowledging the role of masculinities and tailoring interventions accordingly, clinicians can bridge the gap between cultural identity and mental health support. Ultimately, dismantling harmful masculine norms in military and therapeutic contexts is essential to improving PTSD outcomes and restoring psychological well-being in those who have served.

References

Abeyasinghe, N. L., de Zoysa, P., Bandara, K. M. K. C., Bartholameuz, N. A., & Bandara, J. M. U. J. (2012). The prevalence of symptoms of Post-Traumatic Stress Disorder among soldiers with amputation of a limb or spinal injury: A report from a rehabilitation centre in Sri Lanka. *Psychology, Health & Medicine, 17*(3), 376–381.

Akiki, T. J., Averill, C. L., & Abdallah, C. G. (2017). A network-based neurobiological model of PTSD: Evidence from structural and functional neuroimaging studies. *Current Psychiatry Reports, 19*(11), 81.

Alker, Z., & Godfrey, B. (2016). Soldiers and victims: Conceptions of military service and victimhood, 1914–45. In S. Walklate & R. McGarry (Eds.), *The Palgrave handbook of criminology and War* (pp. 133–149). Palgrave Macmillan.

Andrewes, D. G., & Jenkins, L. M. (2019). The role of the frontal lobes in social cognition and executive function in post-traumatic stress disorder. *Brain Sciences, 9*(3), 65.

Bartoli, F., Crocamo, C., Alamia, A., Amidani, F., Paggi, E., Pini, E., Clerici, M., & Carra, G. (2015). Posttraumatic stress disorder and risk of obesity: Systematic review and meta-analysis. *Journal of Clinical Psychiatry, 76*(10), 1253–1261.

Batcho, K. I. (2013). Nostalgia: Retreat or support in difficult times? *American Journal of Psychology, 126*(3), 355–367.

Bliese, P. D., Wright, K. M., Adler, A. B., Cabrera, O., Castro, C. A., & Hoge, C. W. (2011). Validating the primary care posttraumatic stress disorder screen and the posttraumatic stress disorder checklist with soldiers returning from combat. *Journal of Consulting and Clinical Psychology, 76*(2), 272–281.

Brewin, C. R., Garnett, R., & Andrews, B. (2011). Trauma, identity and mental health in UK military veterans. *Psychological Medicine, 41*(8), 1733–1740.

Brock, R. N., & Lettini, G. (2012). *Soul repair: Recovering from moral injury after war*. Beacon Press.

Church, J. (2010). Screening for PTSD in veterans: A review of the literature. *Journal of Nervous and Mental Disease, 198*(12), 882–886.

Connell, R. W. (2016). *Masculinities* (3rd ed.). Polity.

Connell, R. W., & Messerschmidt, J. W. (2005). Hegemonic masculinity: Rethinking the concept. *Gender & Society, 19*(6), 829–859.

Danto, E. A. (2016). Trauma and the state with Sigmund Freud as witness. *International Journal of Law and Psychiatry, 48*, 50–56.

Davidson, P. R., & Parker, K. C. H. (2001). Eye movement desensitization and reprocessing (EMDR): A meta-analysis. *Journal of Consulting and Clinical Psychology, 69*(2), 305–316.

Elbogen, E. B., Wagner, H. R., Johnson, S. C., Kinneer, P. M., Kang, H., Vasterling, J. J., Timko, C., & Beckham, J. C. (2019). Are Iraq and Afghanistan veterans using mental health services? New data from a national survey. *Psychiatric Services, 64*(2), 134–141.

Fitelson, E., Kim, S., Baker, A. S., & Leight, K. (2011). Treatment of postpartum depression: Clinical, psychological, and social perspectives. *International Journal of Women's Health, 3*, 1–14.

Forbes, D., Creamer, M., Phelps, A., et al. (2012). Treating adults with acute stress disorder and PTSD in general practice: A clinical update. *Medical Journal of Australia, 196*(1), 4–11.

French, L. M., McCrea, M., & Baggett, M. (2020). The military acute concussion evaluation: A brief tool to assess traumatic brain injury. *Military Medicine, 185*(5–6), 271–277.

Freud, S. (2016). *Introductory lectures on psychoanalysis*. Routledge (Original work published 1917).

Hurley, E. (2018). Masculinity and military culture in therapy for combat PTSD. *Journal of Contemporary Psychotherapy, 48*(4), 199–207.

Jones, E., & Wessely, S. (2003). "Forward psychiatry" in the military: Its origins and effectiveness. *Journal of Traumatic Stress, 16*(4), 411–419.

Karlin, B. E., Ruzek, J. I., Chard, K. M., Eftekhari, A., Monson, C. M., Hembree, E. A., & Resick, P. A. (2010). Dissemination of evidence-based treatments for PTSD in the Veterans Health Administration. *Journal of Traumatic Stress, 23*(6), 663–673.

Kinghorn, W. A. (2015). Combat trauma and moral fragmentation: A theological account of moral injury. *Journal of the Society of Christian Ethics, 35*(2), 57–74.

Leeb, S. (2018). Freud's theories of war neurosis revisited. *History of Psychiatry, 29*(1), 3–19.

Levandoski, L. A. (2010). Abram Kardiner and the psychoanalytic origins of PTSD. *Psychoanalytic Review, 97*(3), 407–426.

Loughran, T. (2012). *Shell shock and medical culture in First World War Britain*. Cambridge University Press.

MacManus, D., Dean, K., Jones, M., Rona, R. J., Greenberg, N., Hull, L., & Fear, N. T. (2012). Violent offending by UK military personnel deployed to Iraq and Afghanistan: A data linkage cohort study. *Lancet, 380*(9850), 915–921.

Maxfield, L., & Hyer, L. (2002). The relationship between efficacy and methodology in studies investigating EMDR treatment of PTSD. *Journal of Clinical Psychology, 58*(1), 23–41.

Mitchell, J. M., Bogenschutz, M., Lilienstein, A., et al. (2021). MDMA-assisted therapy for severe PTSD: A randomized, double-blind, placebo-controlled Phase 3 study. *Nature Medicine, 27*(6), 1025–1033.

Monson, C. M., Schnurr, P. P., Resick, P. A., Friedman, M. J., Young-Xu, Y., & Stevens, S. P. (2006). Cognitive processing therapy for veterans with military-related posttraumatic stress disorder. *Journal of Consulting and Clinical Psychology, 74*(5), 898–907.

Mulherkar, S., & Tolias, K. F. (2020). RhoA-ROCK signalling as a therapeutic target in traumatic brain injury. *Cells, 9*(1), 245.

Murphy, D., Spencer-Harper, L., Carson, C., Palmer, E., Hill, K., Sorfleet, N., & Busuttil, W. (2016). Long-term responses to treatment in UK veterans with military-related PTSD: An observational study. *BMJ Open, 6*(9), e011473.

Oppizzi, L. M., & Umberger, R. (2018). The use of exercise to manage PTSD symptoms. *Military Medicine, 183*(5–6), e219–e226.

Owens, G. P., Steger, M. F., Whitesell, A. A., & Herrera, C. J. (2012). Posttraumatic stress disorder, guilt, depression, and meaning in life in veterans. *Journal of Traumatic Stress, 22*(3), 254–257.

Passie, T. (2018). The early use of MDMA in psychotherapy (1977–1985). *Drug Science, Policy and Law, 4*(1), 1–13.

Raskind, M. A., Peterson, K., Williams, T., et al. (2013). A trial of prazosin for combat trauma PTSD with nightmares in active-duty soldiers. *American Journal of Psychiatry, 170*(9), 1003–1010.

Ross, J., Armour, C., & Busuttil, W. (2018). The relationship between masculinity and posttraumatic stress disorder in veterans: A latent class analysis. *Psychology of Men & Masculinity, 19*(3), 412–423.

Sharif, K., Watad, A., Bragazzi, N. L., Lichtbroun, M., Amital, H., & Shoenfeld, Y. (2018). Physical activity and autoimmune diseases: Get moving and manage the disease. *Autoimmunity Reviews, 17*(1), 53–72.

Singh, R., Ali, A., & Agarwal, P. (2018). Pharmacotherapy of PTSD: Current status and future directions. *Expert Opinion on Pharmacotherapy, 19*(10), 1057–1068.

Smith, R. T., Masuhara, E. J., & Frueh, B. C. (2014). Nostalgia, Irritable Heart, and Soldier's Heart: PTSD and the evolution of diagnostic constructs. *History of Psychiatry, 25*(2), 139–155.

Valiente-Gómez, A., Moreno-Alcázar, A., Treen, D., Cedrón, C., Colom, F., Pérez, V., & Amann, B. L. (2017). EMDR beyond PTSD: A systematic literature review. *Frontiers in Psychology, 8*, 1668.

Van der Kolk, B. A. (1994). The body keeps the score: Memory and the evolving psychobiology of posttraumatic stress. *Harvard Review of Psychiatry, 1*(5), 253–265.

Varker, T., Watson, L., Forbes, D., et al. (2021). Efficacy of MDMA-assisted psychotherapy for PTSD: Systematic review and meta-analysis. *Journal of Anxiety Disorders, 85*, 102494.

Wampold, B. E., Imel, Z. E., Laska, K. M., et al. (2010). Determining what works in the treatment of PTSD. *Clinical Psychology Review, 30*(7), 923–933.

Williston, S. K., Roos, C. R., & Mannix, L. J. (2020). Mindfulness-based interventions for PTSD among veterans. *Mindfulness, 11*(5), 1083–1096.

Yehuda, R., Vermetten, E., McFarlane, A. C., & Lehrner, A. (2014). PTSD in the military: Special considerations for understanding prevalence, pathophysiology and treatment following deployment. *European Journal of Psychotraumatology, 5*(1), 25322.

CHAPTER 3

Masculinities, Physical Exercise, and PTSD

Mental health problems for military veterans are numerous, with PTSD being a significant concern (Kopacz et al., 2016; Van Gelderen et al., 2018). In order to cater to the diverse range of abilities and preferences that individuals possess, this chapter has included multiple types of exercises. These exercises delve into the topic of PTSD and explore what the latest research has to say about it. By doing so, they not only provide valuable insights into the condition but also help individuals better understand their own experiences (Davidson & Parker, 2001; Najavits, 2002).

However, it's important to acknowledge that these exercises do have drawbacks and limitations (Danto, 2016; Van Gelderen et al., 2018). As with any research, the findings presented here are not without their own biases and may not necessarily apply to every individual (Service, 2009). Nonetheless, by Engaging in these exercises, individuals can gain a better understanding of the nature of PTSD and how it impacts their lives (Ehlers et al., 2005; Monson et al., 2009; Rosenbaum et al., 2015).

The symptoms of PTSD can disrupt various aspects of veterans' lives, including family relationships, social connections, and work performance (Celano et al., 2016; Brewin et al., 2017). When it comes to aerobic activities, research has shown that they often lead to positive physiological changes. However, it's important to examine each activity individually, as there are unique aspects to each one that go beyond just the physical benefits. For instance, swimming has been found to have the added benefit of

J. Alder, *Military Men, Physical Exercise, and Post-Traumatic Stress Disorder*, Palgrave Studies in Masculinity, Sport and Exercise,
https://doi.org/10.1007/978-3-032-08957-1_3

weightlessness, which creates a sense of freedom and relaxation for many individuals (Price et al., 2015; Ross et al., 2018).

On the other hand, hiking might trigger images of traumatic firefights in agrarian areas for some indiv ssing (Asmundson et al., 2013; Elbogen et al., 2019). It is for such reasons that this chapter summaries popular aerobic activities, what the research says about them, as well as their limitations. By doing so, individuals can make more informed decisions about which activities to engage in, and they can also better understand the potential benefits and drawbacks of each (Diaz & Motta, 2008).

Physical exercise has gained increasing recognition as a potential treatment for PTSD symptoms (Caddick & Smith, 2014; Foote et al., 2015). In fact, it has shown promise in not only addressing issues specific to PTSD but also improving overall physical and mental health. Research indicates that physical exercise can effectively alleviate various PTSD symptoms, including anxiety, low mood, hypervigilance, irritability, and nightmares (Broman-Fulks et al., 2004; Finley, 2011; Caddick & Smith, 2018).

Regular physical exercise has been found to have profound effects on the brain. It triggers the release of endorphins, hormones associated with happiness and pain relief. Additionally, exercise activates the hippocampus, a key brain region responsible for memory formation and spatial navigation (Colcombe et al., 2006; Björkman & Ekblom, 2022). The activation of the hippocampus through physical exercise holds significant potential in the context of treating PTSD symptoms, as it plays a crucial role in memory processing.

These findings highlight the importance of physical exercise as a complementary treatment option for individuals with PTSD (Caddick & Smith, 2018; Feduccia & Mithoefer, 2018; Foa et al., 2018). Further research is warranted to deepen our understanding of the specific mechanisms underlying the benefits of exercise in PTSD symptom management and to explore the optimal types and duration of exercise interventions for different populations.

In exploring the correlation between exercise intervention and PTSD, the works of scholars such as Van der Kolk shed light on the intricate relationship between trauma recovery and the body's response to stress (Van der Kolk, 2001). Van der Kolk's research underscores the importance of the brain-body connection in comprehending and treating PTSD (Van der Kolk, 2015). His studies highlight how traumatic experiences can become embodied, resulting in dysregulation of the body's stress response systems. Moreover, Van der Kolk emphasises the role of physical interventions, like exercise, in addressing these bodily manifestations of trauma.

Exercise has been demonstrated to modulate stress hormones, promote neuroplasticity, and regulate the autonomic nervous system, all crucial components in the recovery process from PTSD (Van der Kolk, 1994).

Van der Kolk (2015) suggests that exercise plays a significant role in understanding the modulation of stress hormones among veterans with PTSD, paramount in realising its therapeutic potential. Studies consistently reveal that engaging in regular physical activity can lead to substantial alterations in stress hormone levels, particularly cortisol, pivotal in the body's response to stress (Schöner et al., 2017; Karlin et al., 2010; Van der Kolk, 2006). For veterans grappling with the aftermath of trauma, dysregulated cortisol levels are frequently implicated in exacerbating PTSD symptoms (Van der Kolk, 2003).

This modulation is believed to occur through a combination of factors, including the activation of the hypothalamic-pituitary-adrenal (HPA) axis during exercise and the subsequent release of endorphins, which act as natural stress relievers (Van der Kolk, 2015). Additionally, aerobic exercises such as jogging or cycling have been shown to promote a phenomenon known as "exercise-induced stress adaptation", wherein the body becomes more resilient to stress over time (Caddick & Smith, 2014; Van der Kolk, 1994). By elucidating the intricate relationship between exercise and stress hormone modulation, researchers are paving the way for targeted exercise interventions tailored to the unique needs of veterans with PTSD (Van der Kolk, 2001). These findings underscore the importance of incorporating physical activity into PTSD treatment protocols, offering a holistic approach to symptom management that addresses both the psychological and physiological aspects of PTSD (Van der Kolk, 2015).

Furthermore, as researchers delve deeper into the connections between exercise and trauma recovery, they are exploring how different forms of exercise, including aerobic and anaerobic modalities, can be tailored to address specific PTSD symptoms (Frontera et al., 2006). For instance, studies have demonstrated that aerobic exercises like jogging or cycling not only modulate stress hormones such as cortisol but also promote neuroplasticity, the brain's ability to reorganise and form new neural connections, which is crucial for adapting to and recovering from trauma (Nowacka-Chmielewska et al., 2022). Similarly, anaerobic activities like weightlifting or sprinting have been found to regulate the autonomic nervous system, aiding individuals in better Managing physiological responses to stress and promoting a sense of control and empowerment (Caddick & Smith, 2018; Hegberg et al., 2019). By comprehending the specific effects of each exercise modality on stress physiology and neural processes, researchers can tailor exercise prescriptions to target specific PTSD symptoms effectively, offering personalised approaches to trauma recovery (Nowacka-Chmielewska et al., 2022; Van der Kolk, 2015).

Examining the role of exercise in elucidating the modulation of stress hormones among veterans with PTSD extends beyond the scope of Van der Kolk's research to incorporate the insights of Levine (Levine, 2010). While Van der Kolk's work underscores the importance of the brain-body connection in trauma recovery, Levine's somatic experiencing approach delves deeper into how unresolved trauma manifests in the body and how it can be released through physiological interventions (Levine, 2010; Van der Kolk, 2015). Moreover, research by Levine suggests that trauma can become trapped in the body, leading to chronic stress and dysregulation of the autonomic nervous system (Levine, 2010). In this context, exercise serves as a potent tool for discharging accumulated tension and restoring balance to the nervous system (Levine, 1997).

Studies into Levine's somatic experiencing techniques alongside structured exercise regimes reveal intriguing overlaps (Payne et al., 2015). Both approaches acknowledge the body's innate capacity to heal and adapt, emphasising the importance of physical interventions in trauma recovery (Levine, 2010; Van der Kolk, 2015). Furthermore, findings suggest that exercises targeting proprioceptive awareness and grounding techniques align closely with Levine's principles of somatic experiencing, promoting a sense of safety and embodiment crucial for trauma resolution (Minton et al., 2006).

In terms of stress hormone modulation, while Van der Kolk's research highlights the impact of exercise on cortisol levels and the HPA axis, Levine's work complements this by addressing the broader autonomic nervous system dysregulation observed in PTSD (Levine, 2010; Van der Kolk, 2015). Exercise interventions tailored to incorporate Levine's somatic experiencing principles may offer a holistic approach to trauma recovery, targeting both the psychological and physiological aspects of PTSD (Hoge et al., 2007; Singh et al., 2018). By integrating insights from both Van der Kolk and Levine, researchers are better equipped to develop comprehensive exercise protocols that address the multifaceted nature of trauma, offering new avenues for tailored interventions in PTSD treatment (Hoge et al., 2007; Levine, 2010; Van der Kolk, 2015).

Many physical exercise activities, such as group fitness classes or team sports, provide a sense of community and social support that can have a positive impact on mental health (Asmundson et al., 2013). Engaging in physical exercise with others can create a sense of belonging and connection, which is especially important for individuals who may feel isolated or disconnected from others (Rosenbaum et al., 2015). The shared experience of physical activity can also promote feelings of empathy, teamwork, and motivation (Caddick & Smith, 2018). Furthermore, group exercise can provide a sense of accountability and motivation to maintain a consistent exercise routine (Hegberg et al. 2019). By providing a supportive environment, physical exercise activities can not only improve physical health but also enhance mental and emotional well-being (Hegberg et al. 2019).

The best exercise Programme for armed forces veterans depends on their fitness level, goals, and physical constraints (Hegberg et al. 2019). But exercise, in general, can be broken down into three categories: aerobic, anaerobic, and flexibility training. Each offers various training stimuli and intensities (Mcweeny et al., 2020; Nanclerio et al., 2022), with each category of exercise being performed over a range of moderate to high intensity to be classified as exercise (Cloitre, 2009; Patki et al., 2014).

Aerobic exercises have been found to support and improve cardiovascular fitness and overall health, utilising activities such as Hiking, jogging, cycling, and swimming (American College of Sports Medicine, 2003; Manger & Motta, 2005). Anaerobic exercises are designed to improve muscle strength and power (Cloitre, 2009), utilising activities such as weightlifting and sprinting. Flexibility exercises, including yoga and Pilates, enhance joint range of motion, balance, and posture. In addition to these categories, there are other forms of physical exercises, and many exercises are a hybrid of these three categories (Asmundson et al., 2013).

Researchers continue to argue for and against the merits of anaerobic exercise and the treatment of PTSD in veterans (Arem et al., 2015; Ströhle, 2019). Yet, moderate-intensity aerobic exercise provides significantly more positive psychological impacts than high-intensity aerobic exercise or anaerobic activity, according to Shamus and Cohen's 2009 research. As a result, this chapter will explore the literature on anaerobic exercise, including weightlifting, powerlifting, and other types of aerobic and anaerobic exercise, as a viable therapy for treating PTSD in veterans (Caddick & Smith, 2018; Hegberg et al. 2019).

This chapter delves into the suitability of different forms of physical activity as potential treatments for post-traumatic stress disorder (PTSD) in military veterans. Research studies have consistently demonstrated that veterans who engage in aerobic or anaerobic physical exercise for 0.5 hours per week or weightlifting for 0.25 hours per week experience significantly reduced levels of anxiety and depression compared to veterans who do not engage in any form of physical exercise (Caddick & Smith, 2014).

Furthermore, a substantial body of literature supports the effectiveness of physical exercise in alleviating PTSD symptoms, including anxiety and depression, not only among veterans but also in the general population (Rosenbaum et al., 2015; Schuma, 2016; Shields et al., 2017). This growing body of evidence highlights the significance of physical exercise as a viable treatment option for PTSD, with numerous studies consistently demonstrating its positive impact.

Moreover, ongoing research has explored the mechanisms underlying the effectiveness of physical exercise, revealing insights into how it positively affects neuroplasticity and stress response regulation (Smith et al., 2017; Jones et al., 2020), among other factors.

However, it is crucial to note that not all veterans experience PTSD symptoms similarly, and individual suitability for physical exercise may vary (Diaz & Motta, 2008; Patki et al., 2014; Winett & Ogletree, 2019). Therefore, this chapter aims to explore various types of physical exercises to assess their suitability as potential treatments for military veterans with PTSD. By critically examining the benefits and limitations of physical exercise as a complementary treatment, the chapter seeks to contribute to the development of evidence-based exercise interventions that effectively address the unique needs of veterans with PTSD.

Aerobic Exercise

Aerobic exercise or endurance exercise is defined as physical activity that causes a sustained increase in heart rate and respiration (McArdle, Katch, & Katch, 2010). During this exercise, the body uses oxygen to create energy and maintain motion (Anderson & Shivakumar, 2013; Crombie et al., 2023). According to Asmundson et al. (2013), aerobic exercise includes jogging, brisk walking, swimming, cycling, dancing, and aerobics classes. Additionally, these exercises can be done at different intensities depending on a person's fitness level and goals (Asmundson et al., 2013).

To get the most out of aerobic exercise, it is advised to perform moderate-intensity aerobic activity for at least 150 minutes each week, or 30 minutes each day, five days a week (Asmundson et al., 2013; Patel et al., 2017). Moreover, Asmundson et al. (2013) recommends vigorous-intensity aerobic activity for at least 75 minutes each week for even more significant health benefits, such as, improved cardiovascular health, enhanced respiratory function, and mental well-being. It is recommended for people of all ages and fitness levels to engage in this sort of exercise because it is a crucial part of living a healthy lifestyle (Hupin et al., 2015; Patel et al., 2017). For adults to maintain optimal cardiovascular health, the World Health Organization (WHO) recommends Engaging in at least 150 minutes of aerobic exercise with moderate intensity or 75 minutes of vigorous-intensity aerobic activity per week (Connell & Messerschmidt, 2005).

According to McArdle et al. (2010), aerobic exercise involves the continuous and rhythmic contraction of large muscle groups to burn oxygen for energy. Furthermore, "aerobic" literally means "with oxygen" and refers to the metabolic process by which the body burns fats and carbohydrates to produce energy when oxygen is present (Kraemer et al., 2004).

The body's need for oxygen rises during aerobic exercise, increasing heart rate, breathing rate, and blood flow to the working muscles (McArdle et al., 2010; Patel et al., 2017). Furthermore, the enhanced oxygen delivery enhances fitness and endurance by enabling the muscles to operate more effectively and efficiently (McArdle et al., 2010). Numerous health advantages of aerobic exercise include lowering the risk of chronic illnesses, including diabetes, heart disease, and stroke, enhancing mood and cognitive function, and promoting weight loss and management (Connell, 2016; Bestha et al., 2018).

It is essential to include aerobic exercise in a comprehensive fitness Programme that includes walking and running (O'Donovan et al., 2010). In addition, O'Donovan et al. (2010) found that a fitness Programme that includes weight training, flexibility exercises, balance drills, walking, running, and swimming is important for overall health and well-being. This is because weight training can help to improve bone density, increase muscle mass, and improve metabolism, which can in turn lead to greater calorie burn even at rest (Whitworth et al., 2019). Additionally, when it comes to aerobic exercise, various methods such as heart rate, personal effort, and metabolic equivalent (MET) values can be used to determine the intensity of the exercise (McArdle et al., 2010). Therefore, incorporating weight training in a comprehensive fitness Programme can be a crucial element for overall health and fitness.

The physiological effects of aerobic exercise on the body are extensive and include everything from changes in metabolism and immunological response to adaptations in the cardiovascular system (McArdle et al., 2010). Moreover, McArdle et al. (2010) found acute consequences of aerobic exercise include increased cardiac output, heart rate, stroke volume, and oxygen transport to working muscles. In addition, several adjustments are required to satisfy the body's increased energy requirements during exercise (McArdle et al., 2010; Williamson et al., 2013).

Additionally, during aerobic exercise, the body uses its glycogen stores, or glucose, which are kept in the muscles and liver after being created through a procedure known as glycolysis which provides energy to the brain and supporting various brain functions (McArdle et al., 2010). Moreover, when glycogen is broken down by glycolysis into glucose, this is further changed into a substance known as pyruvate (McArdle et al., 2010). Pyruvate is then broken down in the mitochondria of the cell through a process of chemical reactions, this produces the primary source of energy for cellular processes, Adenosine Triphosphate (ATP), contributing to better diabetes control and lower complication risks (McArdle et al., 2010; Patel et al., 2017).

Another benefit of aerobic exercise is increased endurance (McArdle et al., 2010). This is because regular aerobic exercise can expand the size and number of the mitochondria, which are the cells' energy-producing organelles (Kraemer et al., 2004). As a result, the body can generate more energy while consuming less oxygen, resulting in increased endurance and decreased fatigue during physical activity (McArdle et al., 2010; Patel et al., 2017).

Another physiological result of aerobic exercise is an increase in the number and size of mitochondria, which produce energy in cells (Patel et al., 2017). Due to the body's increased ability to produce energy while consuming less oxygen, physical activity can be performed for extended periods without feeling as tired (Patel et al., 2017).

Additionally, Borghi-Silva et al. (2009) found aerobic exercise can benefit respiratory health. Regular exercise may reduce the risk of developing respiratory conditions like chronic obstructive pulmonary disease (COPD) and improve overall respiratory function by increasing lung capacity and effectiveness (Borghi-Silva et al., 2009).

Regular aerobic exercise is good for the metabolism and the body's composition. Lowering body fat and building muscle can enhance body composition and general health. Additionally, regular exercise can improve insulin sensitivity, allowing the body to regulate blood sugar levels better and lower the risk of type 2 diabetes (Roy et al., 2010).

Regular aerobic exercise causes the cardiovascular system to adapt over time, resulting in changes to the heart's size and strength, blood vessels' number and size, blood pressure, and resting heart rate (McArdle et al., 2010; Patel et al., 2017). Moreover, by enhancing the cardiovascular system's effectiveness, these adaptations enable a more extensive delivery of oxygen and nutrients to the working muscles and a more effective removal of waste materials like carbon dioxide and lactic acid.

Aerobic exercise improves cardiovascular responses and significantly changes metabolic function, leading to enhanced endurance, increased calorie expenditure, and improved overall physical fitness (Sawka, 2011). The body uses carbohydrates and fats as its primary energy sources during training, with each fuel source's proportionate contribution varying with the activity's intensity and length (Sawka, 2011). Therefore, regular aerobic exercise increases the body's capacity to utilise fat as a fuel source, which is advantageous for Managing weight and maintaining general health (Roy et al., 2010). Additionally, aerobic activity increases the quantity and size of mitochondria, the body's energy-producing organelles, which boosts energy production efficiency even more.

Regular aerobic activity increases the body's capacity to utilise fat as a fuel source, which is advantageous for Managing weight and maintaining general health (Wing & Hill, 2001). Additionally, Patel et al. (2017) found aerobic exercise increases the quantity and size of mitochondria, the body's energy-producing organelles, which boosts energy production efficiency even more.

Additionally, aerobic exercise has significant benefits for the immune system. High-intensity activity can momentarily inhibit the immune system (Jee, 2016). However, moderate aerobic exercise has been found to boost immunological function (Patel et al., 2017). In addition, regular aerobic exercise can enhance immune function and lower inflammation, lowering the risk of developing certain illnesses and conditions like cancer and autoimmune disorders (Sharif et al., 2018).

Bone health is another crucial physiological effect of aerobic exercise (Plowman & Smith, 2013). Walking and running are weight-bearing aerobic exercises that help maintain and improve bone density, lowering the risk of osteoporosis and fractures later in life (Plowman & Smith, 2013). Additionally, aerobic activity can increase joint flexibility and decrease the likelihood of joint discomfort and stiffness.

Finally, aerobic activity dramatically affects the brain and mental health (Folkins & Sime, 1981; Mikkelsen et al., 2017). Regular aerobic exercise has been demonstrated to enhance cognitive abilities such as memory, attention, and processing speed. Additionally, aerobic exercise increases the body's natural feel-good chemicals, endorphins, which can elevate mood and lessen the signs of sadness and anxiety.

As a result, aerobic exercise has a variety of physiological consequences on the human body, such as adaptations to the heart, modifications to the metabolism and immune system, enhancements to bone health, and beneficial effects on the brain and mental well-being (Folkins & Sime, 1981; Tsukamoto et al., 2016). Furthermore, acute and chronic adjustments can positively impact one's health and well-being (Mikkelsen et al., 2017). Therefore, individuals with PTSD should incorporate aerobic activity into a balanced fitness Programme for optimum health and well-being.

Aerobic Exercise as a PTSD Treatment

Aerobic physical exercise has been identified as a viable alternative therapy for mental health issues, including depression and PTSD (De Vries et al., 2012). Low-impact aerobic activity has provided veterans with an alternative approach to treating PTSD (Gates et al., 2012). Aerobic exercise predominantly uses the aerobic energy system or relies on oxygen to produce energy and helps reduce symptoms of PTSD, such as anxiety and depression (Kraemer et al., 2004; Ströhle, 2007). It can also improve sleep quality and minimise hyperarousal.

Aerobic exercise has several advantages that benefit cardiovascular and mental health. By increasing the effectiveness of the heart and lungs, it improves cardiovascular health (Kraemer et al., 2004). It also provides more oxygen to the muscles during exercise, enabling them to function more effectively, resulting in more energy, improved stamina, a lower risk of developing cardiovascular disease, as well as supporting mental health (Kraemer et al., 2004).

Moreover, aerobic exercise boosts metabolism and burns calories, which helps people lose weight and become more insulin-sensitive, lowering the chance of developing type 2 diabetes (Roy et al., 2010). Reducing the risk of type 2 diabetes and improving metabolism support the reduction of mental health symptoms like anxiety disorders (Roy et al., 2010).

Aerobic exercise positively affects the hypothalamic-pituitary-adrenal (HPA) axis, which controls the body's stress response system (McArdle et al., 2010). Participation in a structured aerobic exercise Programme led to individuals living with PTSD displaying improvements in the health of their HPA axis and decreased levels of the stress hormone cortisol (Hegberg et al., 2019). Despite such findings, researchers do not fully understand how aerobic exercise may reduce PTSD symptoms (Ley et al., 2018).

Several theories have been put forward, such as physical activity boosting the production of endorphins, which act as natural opioids to soothe pain, improve well-being, and reduce PTSD symptoms (Mikkelsen et al., 2017). Exercise may also aid in controlling the HPA axis, which is responsible for the stress response (Popovic et al., 2022). Additionally, exercise has been demonstrated to enhance sleep quality, which may be advantageous for people with PTSD who frequently have sleep difficulties (Ströhle, 2019).

Moderate-intensity cardiovascular activities, such as brisk walking, hiking, cycling, or swimming, have been shown to alleviate symptoms associated with PTSD potentially (Asmundson et al., 2013). These exercises are convenient for many people as they are not too strenuous and can be easily incorporated into daily activities (Bestha et al., 2018; Hegberg et al., 2019). Additionally, studies have suggested that moderate-intensity aerobic training may improve mood and reduce stress (Whitworth & Ciccolo, 2016; Bestha et al., 2018). Moderate-intensity aerobic exercise has also been found to potentially decrease symptoms of anxiety and depression and improve sleep quality in individuals with PTSD (Asmundson et al., 2013; Bestha et al., 2018). Therefore, this section focuses on the potential relationship between aerobic exercise and symptoms associated with PTSD.

Aerobic Exercise and PTSD Symptomology

Walking is a form of aerobic exercise that can be performed at brisk speeds, falling within the range of aerobic activity (Bichler et al., 2022). It is a well-known and accessible method for improving overall health and fitness, as it can be done at any time and in any location (Asmundson et al., 2013; Hall et al., 2016). Veterans with PTSD may find walking particularly beneficial in Managing their condition, as suggested by Vancampfort et al. (2017). Notably, regular walking has been associated with a 50% decrease in PTSD symptoms, as reported by Asmundson et al. (2013). Additionally, individuals who engage in 30 minutes of daily walking experience an increase in positive emotions like happiness and joy, along with a decrease in negative emotions such as fear and anger (Asmundson et al., 2013; Legarreta et al., 2015).

Research also highlights the positive impact of walking on sleep quality, a crucial aspect for individuals with PTSD who often suffer from sleep disturbances. Walking has been shown to improve sleep quality (Cordier et al., 2019) and reduce stress levels, while concurrently enhancing self-esteem in individuals with PTSD (Stubbs et al., 2017; Hall & Knuth, 2019).

Nevertheless, it is important to recognise potential drawbacks associated with walking for individuals with PTSD. Strenuous walking may trigger flashbacks or intrusive memories related to combat experiences (Bremner & Marmar, 2002; Collins & Long, 2003). In contrast, engaging in slower, relaxing walks may create a safer environment unrelated to combat (Collins & Long, 2003). Adherence to a walking routine might pose challenges for individuals with PTSD due to motivation or energy issues (Stern et al., 2013). Furthermore, physical disabilities that limit walking ability need to be taken into account (Bremner & Marmar, 2002; Collins & Long, 2003; Stern et al., 2013).

Hiking

Hiking is a form of aerobic exercise that distinguishes itself from walking by being performed on challenging natural terrains such as trails, steep inclines, and uneven surfaces, often over longer distances. This physically demanding activity is an effective way to enhance overall health and fitness (Nisenbaum et al., 2000; Oppizzi & Umberger, 2018). In addition to the physical benefits, hiking offers numerous mental advantages, such as reducing anxiety and hypervigilance. By immersing oneself in nature, hiking provides a calming effect, promotes the release of exercise-induced endorphins, encourages mindfulness and grounding, exposes individuals to stress-reducing green spaces, fosters social connections, and offers cognitive stimulation and distraction from anxious thoughts (Lackey et al., 2021).

Recent research has shown that hiking can effectively reduce symptoms of anxiety, depression, and improve overall physical well-being (Bettmann et al., 2021; Bryan et al., 2018). It has also been associated with improved sleep quality, stress reduction, and enhanced self-esteem (Davis-Berman et al., 2018; Lackey et al., 2021). However, it is worth noting that some veterans have reported negative experiences with hiking, particularly when uphill slopes evoke memories of their military service (Burke & Utley, 2013).

While recent studies have explored the potential benefits of hiking in treating PTSD symptoms (Nisenbaum et al., 2000; Oppizzi & Umberger,

2018), more research is needed to establish its effectiveness. Regular hiking Programmes have been found to decrease symptoms of anxiety, depression, and enhance overall well-being (Bettmann et al., 2021). Furthermore, hiking has demonstrated significant reductions in anxiety, depression, and low mood among individuals with PTSD (Bryan et al., 2018). It has also been linked to improved sleep quality, stress reduction, and enhanced self-esteem (Davis-Berman et al., 2018; Lackey et al., 2021).

Despite the potential benefits, it is important to acknowledge some potential drawbacks of hiking as a treatment for PTSD, as suggested by Bettmann et al. (2016).

The strenuous nature of hiking can potentially trigger traumatic flashbacks or intrusive memories in individuals with PTSD who have experienced life-threatening situations or gunfire (Bremner & Marmar, 2002; Collins & Long, 2003). However, choosing less demanding hiking routes can provide a safer environment and reduce the risk of triggering PTSD symptoms (Collins & Long, 2003). Additionally, individuals with PTSD may struggle with adhering to a hiking routine due to lack of focus, motivation, or energy (Stern et al., 2013). Furthermore, physical disabilities may limit hiking accessibility as a treatment option (Bremner & Marmar, 2002; Stern et al., 2013). Thus, further research is needed to better understand the effectiveness of hiking as a treatment for PTSD (Davis-Berman et al., 2018; Lackey et al., 2021).

In conclusion, while some studies suggest the potential benefits of hiking as a treatment for PTSD, more research is required to fully understand its efficacy (Bettmann et al., 2016). It is important to note that hiking may not be suitable for all individuals with PTSD, as specific terrains, environments, or actions may trigger or exacerbate symptoms (Bremner & Marmar, 2002; Collins & Long, 2003). Additionally, previous studies have limitations, such as small sample sizes, which can lead to differing results (Davis-Berman et al., 2018). Therefore, more comprehensive research is necessary to assess the suitability of hiking as a potential treatment option for veterans with PTSD.

Swimming

Swimming is an aerobic exercise that involves moving through water by utilising swimming strokes, including freestyle, breaststroke, backstroke, and butterfly (Stallman, 2017). Swimming is a low-impact exercise that can provide a full-body workout to improve cardiovascular health, build endurance and strength (Brackley et al., 2020). In addition, swimming is accessible to people of all abilities and can be performed in various environments, including pools and open water, for recreational and competitive swimming events (Brackley et al., 2020; Eckstrom et al., 2020). Lastly, swimming has been widely used as part of a therapy routine for people with disabilities and injury recovery (Cooper & Quatrano, 1999).

When prescribing swimming, consider individuals' fitness level, goals, and health (Stern et al., 2013). Begin with once a week and progress to 2–3 times/week for cardio fitness. Start with 20–30 minutes, then increase to 45+ minutes, maintaining a steady pace and gradually increasing effort (Price et al., 2015). Vary distances, starting with 10–20 lengths (250–500m) and working towards 30+ lengths (750m+). Incorporate any of the four recognised swimming strokes (breaststroke, backstroke, butterfly, and front crawl) to improve balance, engage muscles, and prevent injuries (Cole et al., 2022).

Swimming has been found to benefit individuals with PTSD, as suggested by Price et al. (2015). They propose that weightlessness in swimming can reduce symptoms of PTSD, including stress, anxiety, and depression. This effect is attributed to the relaxation response triggered by water's soothing effect, sensory stimulation, endorphin release during exercise, the distraction and mastery provided by swimming, and the social connection and support gained from participating in swimming activities. Additionally, swimming has been associated with improving mood, reducing anxiety, depression, and stress, enhancing social connectedness, improving quality of life, and promoting better sleep (Foote et al., 2015; Price et al., 2015). It has been reported that swimming is a practical and relaxing intervention for individuals with complex PTSD symptoms, particularly after using established traditional therapies (Bernard et al., 2021).

Arem et al. (2015) suggest aerobic exercise, particularly swimming, has been shown to provide a feasible and practical approach to PTSD with individuals experiencing improved sleep and eating habits and a reduction of anxiety and stress. Also, swimming elicits positive effects on cardiovascular fitness and overall health, coupled with its ability to alleviate the debilitating symptoms of intense psychological distress of recurring memories of traumatic events (Arem et al., 2015).

In addition, swimming has been discovered to be a more effective form of exercise for lowering symptoms of anxiety and melancholy (Patki et al., 2014). Moreover, Bernard et al. (2021) suggest the benefits of swimming for individuals with PTSD include improving deep breathing, reducing muscle tension, and promoting relaxation, leading to improved sleep and anxiety. Additionally, veterans with physical wounds or disabilities due to military service have found swimming significantly beneficial in supporting their physical recovery and Managing PTSD symptoms (Patki et al., 2014). Furthermore, Lloret et al. (2021) discovered that swimming had been proven to reduce anxiety and depression, improve overall mood, and have equally promising signs of Managing traumatic memories.

Despite the evidence for the benefits of swimming in treating PTSD, Cole et al. (2022) suggest some potential drawbacks. First, swimming can be challenging and distressing for weak swimmers and potentially increase the likelihood of worry and tension, leading to heightened stress (Cole et al., 2022).

Additionally, individuals with PTSD may find it challenging to adhere to a swimming Programme due to lacking motivation or energy (Stern et al., 2013). Previous studies on swimming were mostly small-scale and focused solely on the short-term effects, neglecting the long-term benefits (Bremner & Marmar, 2002; Stern et al., 2013). They involved a limited number of participants and failed to explore the extended advantages of swimming. As a result, there is a lack of comprehensive evidence regarding the long-term benefits of swimming.

Overall, the evidence for the efficacy of swimming as a treatment for PTSD is still limited. While several studies have suggested that swimming may be beneficial, more research is needed to determine the full potential of this aerobic activity (Cole et al., 2022).

Additionally, current evidence from studies lacks any long-term efficacy and mechanisms of swimming for PTSD treatment (Lloret et al., 2021). Lastly, studies on swimming were conducted on relatively healthy individuals, which may limit the generalisability of the results to individuals with more severe PTSD symptoms (Bernard et al., 2021; Lloret et al., 2021). Therefore, more detailed research into the potential long-term benefits of swimming is required to assess its suitability in providing a possible treatment option for veterans with PTSD.

Running and Jogging

Running and jogging are both forms of aerobic exercise that involve moving at a faster pace—and are more rigorous than walking or hiking and have long been touted as a fantastic way to get fit and stay healthy (Otto & Smits, 2011; Crombie et al., 2019). Moreover, running is primarily considered to be performed at a faster pace than jogging, but these terms are often used interchangeably (Hall et al., 2016). In addition, this aerobic activity predominantly engages the legs and lower body while employing the core and upper body muscles to maintain balance and stability (McArdle et al., 2010; Patel et al., 2017; Speer et al., 2019).

Running and jogging are prevalent aerobic activities that can be done individually or as a group and performed indoors on a treadmill or outdoors on a track, trail, or road (Asmundson et al., 2013; Hall et al., 2016). Additionally, running or jogging can be modified to accommodate all fitness levels and abilities to improve cardiovascular health, burn calories, and build strength and endurance (McArdle et al., 2010; Patel et al., 2017).

Growing evidence supports running or jogging as a treatment for PTSD, with these aerobic activities being associated with significant improvements in sleep quality and reductions in anxiety (Owens et al., 2012; Oppizzi & Umberger, 2018). Moreover, Rosenbaum et al. (2015) found when individuals with PTSD symptoms completed a 12-week running Programme, they experienced improved cardiovascular health and decreased signs of anxiety and depression. Furthermore, Van der Kolk et al. (2014) suggest that running or jogging routines can help individuals with PTSD regulate their emotions, decrease arousal cues, improve sleep and concentration, and reduce feeling jumpy and easily irritated and angered.

In addition, Van der Kolk et al. (2014) suggest individuals with PTSD who participated in running or jogging for at least 30 minutes per day for at least three weeks had significantly reduced levels of anger, anxiety, and depression compared to those who did not run. Moreover, those who took part in running or jogging as part of a therapeutic overall health routine found benefits for individuals with PTSD, with decreased signs of anxiety and depression (Rosenbaum et al., 2015).

Despite the evidence of the benefits of running or jogging in treating PTSD, it's essential to recognise some drawbacks. First, not all veterans may be physically capable of running, which could limit the accessibility of this therapy for some individuals (Bremner & Marmar, 2002; Stathopoulou et al., 2006). In addition, Paolucci et al. (2018) suggest that high-intensity exercise, such as running, can sometimes worsen symptoms of anxiety and depression, so it may not be suitable for everyone. Moreover, there remains limited research on the long-term effects of running for PTSD treatment, which could affect its efficacy over time (Hall et al., 2016; Markotić et al., 2020). Lastly, previous studies have limitations with small sample sizes, leading to differing results (Davis-Berman et al., 2018). Therefore, more detailed research into the potential benefits of running or jogging is required to assess its suitability in providing a possible treatment option for veterans with PTSD.

Cycling

Cycling is an aerobic activity that involves riding a bicycle and is a low-impact exercise that can be performed at varying intensities (Babson et al., 2015). Cycling is a popular aerobic exercise used for recreational purposes and as a means of transportation or performed in professional and Olympic competitions (Rosenberger et al., 2019; Sadeghi et al., 2022). Moreover, cycling can be done indoors on a stationary bike or outdoors on various surfaces, including roads, trails, and mountainous terrain. It can be performed individually or as a competitive team (Babson et al., 2015).

In addition, cycling primarily engages the legs and lower body muscles when pedalling the bicycle but also activates the core and upper body muscles to help to maintain balance and stability (Babson et al., 2015). Furthermore, cycling is an activity that is accessible to people of all abilities and a great form of aerobic exercise that can improve cardiovascular health, build endurance and strength, as well as burn calories (Bloomer et al., 2005; Ma et al., 2021).

Due to its advantages for cardiovascular health, cycling has become increasingly popular as a recreational activity with individuals with PTSD in recent years (Bettmann et al., 2021). In addition, there is growing evidence that cycling can reduce PTSD symptoms, with individuals with PTSD experiencing improved sleep quality and decreased anxiety and depression (Rosenbaum et al., 2015).

Moreover, Pebole and Hall (2019) found the release of endorphins during bouts of cycling aided veterans in lowering the signs and symptoms of increased arousal, anxiety, and despair. Furthermore, cycling outdoors has proven to foster awareness and a sense of connection with the environment, which has led to a favourable impact on mental health and a reduction in PTSD symptoms such as emotional numbness and avoidance of people and places (Ma et al., 2021).

In addition, Carek et al. (2011) discovered that individuals with PTSD who biked for 30 minutes, three times per week, reported fewer symptoms of anxiety and despair. Moreover, individuals with PTSD who participated in some form of cycling had an increase in self-reported physical activity levels and enhanced mood and decreased anxiety (Babson et al., 2015).

Despite the evidence supporting the benefits of cycling in treating PTSD, it is important to acknowledge and address certain drawbacks: Firstly, while there have been advancements in adapted bicycles for individuals with disabilities, it remains challenging for veterans who lack the physical capability to participate in cycling, thus limiting the accessibility of this therapy (Bremner & Marmar, 2002; Stathopoulou et al., 2006).

Furthermore, the complex symptomology of PTSD, including intense or prolonged psychological distress, can pose obstacles to adopting the comprehensive and interdisciplinary approach required for cycling as a therapy (Brittain & Green, 2012). Additionally, some veterans may be unable to engage in cycling due to physical limitations, such as musculoskeletal injuries, or accessibility concerns related to their environment (Goldstein et al., 2018).

Moreover, it is crucial to recognise that physical activity may not be suitable for all individuals with PTSD, particularly those with co-occurring disorders or specific trauma triggers. This underscores the importance of a more individualised and comprehensive approach to treatment, one that takes into account the unique needs and circumstances of each person (Gurak et al., 2016).

By considering these limitations and tailoring the approach accordingly, it is possible to navigate the challenges associated with cycling as a treatment for PTSD, ensuring that the therapy is both safe and effective for those who can benefit from it (Murphy et al., 2016; Goldstein et al., 2018).

In addition, there's still limited research on the long-term effects of cycling for PTSD treatment, which could affect its efficacy over time (Goldstein et al., 2018). Lastly, one of the main limitations of studies on cycling and PTSD has generally been small sample sizes which significantly impact the results and further limit the efficacy of the impact cycling has on PTSD (Davis-Berman et al., 2018). Therefore, more comprehensive research into the potential benefits of cycling is required to assess its suitability in providing a possible treatment option for veterans with PTSD.

Skipping and Jump Rope

Skipping or jumping rope is an aerobic or recreational activity involving an individual jumping over a rope that is swung individually or by others (Oppizzi & Umberger, 2018). Moreover, skipping or jumping rope requires the individual to jump over the rope whilst holding an end of the rope in each hand, or with the rope being held by others, as the rope swings over the head of the one jumping; and is done repeatedly (Pebole et al., 2022). Furthermore, skipping or jumping rope is a popular aerobic exercise widely used as part of a physical training routine to help improve cardiovascular fitness and agility (Cook, 2003).

There is some evidence in current literature that points to the use of skipping or jump rope as a potential treatment for PTSD, with this aerobic exercise being associated with improvements in sleep and a reduction in anger and depression (Cook, 2003; Oppizzi & Umberger, 2018). Moreover, Oppizzi and Umberger (2018) found that individuals with PTSD symptoms who completed 30 minutes of skipping within their training Programme experienced improved cardiovascular health and reduced symptoms of anxiety, nightmares, intrusive thoughts, and depression. Furthermore, Kirthika et al. (2019) suggest that skipping improves cardio output, enhances physical well-being, aids PTSD individuals in emotional regulation, improves sleep and concentration, and reduces jumpiness, irritability, and anger.

Despite the positive findings in the current literature on the benefits of skipping and jumping rope in treating PTSD, it's essential to recognise some drawbacks. First, not all veterans may be physically capable of skipping, which could limit the accessibility of this form of therapy for some individuals (Goldstein et al., 2018).

In addition, Oppizzi and Umberger (2018) also suggest that high-intensity aerobic exercise, such as skipping, has the potential for adverse effects, such as exercise-induced injury and worsening symptoms of anxiety and depression, so it may not be suitable for everyone. Moreover, there's still limited research on the long-term effects of skipping or jumping rope for PTSD treatment, which could affect its efficacy over time (Davis-Berman et al., 2018; Leeb, 2018). Lastly, previous studies have limitations in sample sizes, leading to differing results (Pebole et al., 2022). Therefore, more detailed research into the potential benefits of skipping or jumping rope is required to assess its suitability in providing a possible treatment option for veterans with PTSD.

Anaerobic Exercise

Anaerobic exercise involves short, high-intensity bursts of physical activity that typically last between 30 seconds and 2 minutes (McArdle et al., 2010; Poole et al., 2021). This type of exercise is characterised by high levels of physical exertion and working at or around maximum effort for brief periods, as described by Patel et al. (2017). Examples of anaerobic exercise include sprinting, weightlifting, plyometrics, callisthenics, and high-intensity interval training (HIIT) (Spurway, 1992).

Anaerobic exercise is advised to perform a high-intensity anaerobic activity, which places significant stress on the muscles and stimulates muscle strength and power (McArdle et al., 2010). Furthermore, Patel et al. (2017) found that muscles adapt and get stronger over time when you regularly put them under high-intensity stress.

In addition, anaerobic exercise is often undertaken in brief, intense bursts of activity lasting only a few seconds to a few minutes, with short rest periods for recovery (Poole et al., 2021). Weightlifting, running, jumping, and other high-intensity interval training are a few examples of anaerobic exercise (Spurway, 1992). Moreover, Tomlin and Wenger (2001) suggest anaerobic exercise can be highly taxing on the body and allow adequate rest and recovery time between intervals. As a result, the body can replenish energy stores and recover from strenuous exercise. Furthermore, planning for good rest and recovery prevents damage and repair and permits muscle growth and anaerobic progression and muscle (Tomlin & Wenger, 2001).

Patel et al. (2017) recommend anaerobic exercise as a crucial component of a healthy lifestyle, suitable for people of all ages and fitness levels. The World Health Organization (WHO) also recommends engaging in at least 150 minutes of moderate exercise or 75 minutes of vigorous-intensity activity per week for optimal cardiovascular health (Patel et al., 2017). To achieve a balanced training routine, it is suggested to include at least two anaerobic exercise sessions in addition to regular aerobic exercise training (Patel et al., 2017).

Physiological Benefits of Anaerobic Exercise

Anaerobic exercise has a wide range of physiological effects on the body, including alterations in metabolism and immune system response and adjustments in the cardiovascular system (McArdle et al., 2010). Moreover, McArdle et al. (2010) found acute consequences of anaerobic exercise include increased heart rate and blood pressure, lactate production, elevated breathing rate, and depletion of energy stores. In addition, to meet the body's increased energy demands during anaerobic exercise, several modifications are also necessary, such as enhanced oxygen uptake, increased muscle strength and power, optimised energy systems, effective recovery and adaptation, and mental resilience. These modifications optimise performance, sustain activity, and promote overall well-being (McArdle et al., 2010; Varker et al., 2021).

Another benefit of anaerobic exercise is accelerating the rate of metabolism and calorie burn owing to its fast, devoid of oxygen, energy production (McArdle et al., 2010). This is because anaerobic exercise increases heart rate and blood pressure, which helps deliver nutrients to the working muscles (McArdle et al., 2010). Moreover, Patel et al. (2017) found bouts of anaerobic exercise can lead to an increase in the rate of metabolism and calorie burn during and after anaerobic exercise. Furthermore, after participating in anaerobic exercise, an increase in metabolic rate and calorie burn will assist with weight loss and better body composition over time (McArdle et al., 2010; Patel et al., 2017).

Additionally, during anaerobic exercise, the contractions of muscles are primarily powered by the synthesis of adenosine triphosphate (ATP), which is produced from stored creatine phosphate and glycogen (McArdle et al., 2010). Moreover, Patel et al. (2017) explain glycogen, a complex carbohydrate stored in the liver and muscles that can be converted into glucose for use as fuel, is a molecule rapidly broken down to produce ATP. In contrast, creatine phosphate is a molecule that can be rapidly converted into ATP (Bessman & Carpenter, 1985).

In addition, when performing anaerobic exercises, the body is required to utilise two energy systems, which are the Adenosine Triphosphate-Phosphocreatine system (ATP-PCR) and the Glycolytic system (Zupan et al., 2009). As previously highlighted, anaerobic exercise doesn't use oxygen for energy, demonstrating the importance of both (ATP-PCR) and Glycolytic systems to perform effectively during physical activities (Zupan et al., 2009). Moreover, Zupan et al. (2009) explain ATP-PCR produces energy without the need for oxygen, but that ATP-PCR stores are limited, are quickly depleted, and only provide up to ten seconds of energy when performing at maximal effort during sprinting or Olympic weightlifting set. While the process of glycolysis yields ATP and lactic acid as by-products, which can result in fatigue and muscle soreness, the glycolytic system produces energy best suited for performing up to two minutes during anaerobic activities, such as a 400-meter sprint or weightlifting for muscle hypertrophy (Lopes-Silva et al., 2018).

Regular anaerobic exercise is good for the improvement of muscular strength, power, and endurance (Zupan et al., 2009). Likewise, anaerobic exercise promotes lowering body fat and building muscle and can enhance body composition and general health. In addition, regular anaerobic exercise can improve insulin sensitivity and glucose metabolism, allowing the body to regulate blood sugar levels better and lower the risk of type 2 diabetes (Sato et al., 2003).

Bone health is another crucial physiological effect of anaerobic exercise (McArdle et al., 2010; Patel et al., 2017). Resistance training and weightlifting are weight-resistant anaerobic exercises that help maintain and improve bone density, lowering the risk of osteoporosis and fractures later in life (Kraemer et al., 2002). Furthermore, regular anaerobic exercise can aid neuromuscular coordination and enhance overall physical performance (Lopes-Silva et al., 2018).

Finally, as a result, anaerobic exercise can positively affect the brain and mental health (Kashihara et al., 2009). Indeed, Kashihara et al. (2009) found anaerobic exercise to enhance cognitive abilities such as memory, attention, and processing speed. Additionally, participation in anaerobic exercise increases the body's natural feel-good chemicals, endorphins, which can elevate mood and lessen the signs of sadness and anxiety (Kashihara et al., 2009; McArdle et al., 2010).

Anaerobic Exercise as a PTSD Treatment

Research into anaerobic exercise is not as extensive as aerobic exercise. However, anaerobic exercise has been identified as a viable alternative therapy for mental health such as anxiety, depression, and PTSD (Zschucke et al., 2013). Moreover, anaerobic exercise may be beneficial in treating PTSD because it improves sleep quality, lowers agitation and depressive symptoms, and boosts self-esteem (Hegberg et al., 2019). Additionally, Smith and Merwin (2021) note how the release of endorphins during high-intensity anaerobic exercise can support the treatment of complex PTSD symptoms, such as avoidance behaviours and negative thoughts (Smith & Merwin, 2021). Furthermore, muscles work harder during high-intensity exercise and have been shown to produce endorphins, which are neurotransmitters in the brain that naturally produce anti-anxiety and anti-pain properties (Martland et al., 2020; Smith & Merwin, 2021).

In addition, Asmundson et al. (2013) suggest the endorphins released due to high-intensity anaerobic exercise aid in decreasing symptoms of stress, anxiety, and depression, which are commonly associated with

PTSD. Moreover, high-intensity anaerobic workouts have been shown to reduce anger, anxiety, and social avoidance (Asmundson et al., 2013).

Anaerobic exercise has been demonstrated to boost the synthesis of additional neurotransmitters, including dopamine and serotonin (Mazzardo-Martins et al., 2010).

Additionally, individuals with PTSD experienced significant improvements in their mood and sleep quality following exposure to a high-intensity anaerobic exercise training Programme (Asmundson et al., 2013). Furthermore, Asmundson et al. (2013) suggest individuals with PTSD who participated in a structured eight-week anaerobic weightlifting Programme showed significant neurobiological improvements and reduced PTSD symptoms, such as anxiety, flashbacks, avoidance behaviours, and hyperarousal.

According to Asmundson et al. (2013), moderate-intensity anaerobic activities such as powerlifting, resistance training, and sprinting, can help ease PTSD symptoms. In addition, these exercises are accessible to many people and adaptable to abilities and fitness goals and are simple to include in daily activities (Kashihara et al., 2009). Moreover, research has revealed that moderate-high intensity anaerobic training has been found to improve mood and relieve stress (Lopes-Silva et al., 2018). Furthermore, high-intensity anaerobic exercise led to decreased symptoms of anxiety and depression and enhanced sleep within individuals with PTSD (Asmundson et al., 2013). Therefore, this section will cover the relationship between anaerobic exercises and PTSD symptomology.

Weightlifting, Powerlifting, and Resistance Training

Weightlifting, powerlifting, and resistance training are all forms of anaerobic exercise that utilise free weights, machines, and bodyweight to enhance muscle strength and size. Weightlifting, which has been an official Olympic event since 1896, is a cost-effective and effective physical training method that improves overall health and fitness (Goldstein et al., 2018). It has been associated with numerous benefits, including better sleep quality, reduced anxiety symptoms, improved self-esteem, and a sense of accomplishment (LeBouthillier & Asmundson, 2017; Whitworth et al., 2019).

While weightlifting holds promise in benefiting individuals with PTSD by reducing anxiety sensitivity and distress tolerance (LeBouthillier & Asmundson, 2017), it may also present challenges for them, such as triggering traumatic memories or facing difficulties with motivation or physical disabilities (Begin et al., 2019). Further exploration is needed to fully understand the benefits and suitability of weightlifting as a treatment option for veterans with PTSD, especially through research involving larger sample sizes (Davis-Berman et al., 2018; Ferrer & Davis, 2019).

Powerlifting, involving the squat, bench press, and deadlift, is another form of anaerobic exercise that is performed at the Olympic Games (Poston et al., 2016). It has shown to enhance mood, reduce anxiety, improve sleep, and boost self-confidence (Ferrer & Davis, 2019; Klimek et al., 2018). Powerlifting may offer advantages in addressing fight, flight, or freeze responses in individuals with PTSD (Björkman & Ekblom, 2022). However, it is important to consider potential drawbacks such as triggering flashbacks, low motivation or energy levels, and limitations for individuals with physical disabilities (Begin et al., 2019).

Resistance training, which encompasses various exercises like weightlifting, bodyweight workouts, and machine exercises, is an effective form of anaerobic exercise as well (Whitworth et al., 2019). It has been associated with improved sleep quality, decreased anxiety and depression symptoms, and increased self-confidence (Crombie et al., 2023; Mikkelsen et al., 2017). Resistance training can also benefit individuals with PTSD by managing fight, flight, or freeze responses and improving distress tolerance (Whitworth et al., 2019; Asmundson et al., 2013). However, it is crucial to consider potential drawbacks, such as triggering traumatic memories, low motivation or energy levels, and physical limitations (Begin et al., 2019; Rosenbaum et al., 2015).

Weightlifting, powerlifting, and resistance training offer various benefits for overall health and fitness (Asmundson et al., 2013). While they show potential in treating PTSD, further research with larger sample sizes is necessary to fully understand their advantages and suitability as treatment options for veterans with PTSD (Begin et al., 2019). By addressing these research gaps and acknowledging the potential challenges, we can better inform individuals with PTSD about the potential benefits and considerations of engaging in these forms of exercise (Davis-Berman et al., 2018; Whitworth et al., 2019).

Sprinting Training

Sprinting is a form of anaerobic exercise that can positively impact physical and mental health (Greist et al., 1979; Pedersen et al., 2017). In addition, sprinting training involves high-intensity running over short distances for bouts typically lasting 30 seconds (Pedersen et al., 2017). Moreover, Wadley and Le Rossignol (1998) point out that sprinting training is being designed to improve an individual's speed, power, and overall athletic performance.

Moreover, Callaghan (2004) discovered that anaerobic activity, such as sprinting training, has been associated with lowering anxiety, hopelessness, and depressive moods, as well as improving cognitive performance and self-esteem. Similarly, individuals with PTSD who engage in sprinting training have improved sleep and self-esteem (Qureshi et al., 2011; Patel et al., 2017).

Sprinting training is a prevalent anaerobic activity that can be done individually or as a group and performed indoors on a treadmill or outdoors on a track (Asmundson et al., 2013; Hall et al., 2016). Additionally, sprinting training can be modified to accommodate all fitness levels and abilities and is found to improve cardiovascular health, burn calories, and build strength and endurance (McArdle et al., 2010; Patel et al., 2017). In addition, this anaerobic activity predominantly engages the legs and lower body while also employing the core and upper body muscles to maintain balance and stability (McArdle et al., 2010; Patel et al., 2017).

Growing evidence supports the use of sprinting training as a treatment for PTSD, with these anaerobic activities being associated with significant improvements in sleep quality and reductions in anxiety (Oppizzi & Umberger, 2018). Moreover, Rosenbaum et al. (2015) found that when individuals with PTSD symptoms completed a structured 12-week sprint training Programme, they experienced improved cardiovascular health and elicited decreased signs of anxiety and depression. Furthermore, Van der Kolk et al. (2014) suggest that sprinting routines can help individuals with PTSD regulate their emotions, decrease avoidance cues, and improve their sleeping and concentration.

In addition, studies on sprinting training with individuals with PTSD found that those who participated between two and three times per week, with 48 hours of rest between sessions, experienced significantly reduced levels of anger, anxiety, and depression compared to those who did not run (Van der Kolk et al., 2014). Moreover, studies into sprinting training as part of a therapeutic overall health routine have found benefits for individuals with PTSD, with decreased signs of anxiety and depression (Rosenbaum et al., 2015).

Despite the evidence for the benefits of sprinting training in treating PTSD, it's essential to recognise some drawbacks. First, not all veterans may be physically capable of sprinting, which could limit the accessibility of this therapy for some individuals (Bremner & Marmar, 2002; Stathopoulou et al., 2006). Paolucci et al. (2018) suggest that high-intensity exercise, such as sprinting, can sometimes worsen symptoms of anxiety and depression due to the release of stress hormones and physiological responses that can exacerbate these conditions, making it unsuitable for some individuals. Moreover, there's still limited research on the long-term effects of sprinting for PTSD treatment, which could affect its efficacy over time (Lucibello et al., 2020; Markotić et al., 2020). Lastly, previous studies have limitations in sample sizes, leading to differing results (Davis-Berman et al., 2018; Martland et al., 2020). Therefore, more detailed research into the potential benefits of sprinting training is required to assess its suitability in providing a possible treatment option for veterans with PTSD.

Plyometrics and Callisthenics

Plyometrics and callisthenics are two forms of anaerobic exercise often used to improve strength, power, and agility (Michailidis et al., 2013). In addition, Ratamess (2021) points to plyometrics as a high-intensity exercise involving quick, explosive movements designed to improve power, speed, and agility. Moreover, Breitbach et al. found that callisthenics exercises use the body's weight and not equipment to provide resistance and are designed to improve strength, endurance, and flexibility. Furthermore, plyometrics and callisthenics are widely performed to improve physical performance and have been linked with reduced symptoms of anxiety (Groer et al., 2015; Hegberg et al., 2019).

In addition, plyometrics and callisthenics are growing in popularity as a form of anaerobic exercise, and are utilised to improve agility, strength, and endurance, leading to improved sleep quality (Groer et al., 2015). Moreover, Breitbach et al. found plyometrics and callisthenics engage bodyweight movements to improve cardiovascular fitness and athletic performance, leading to decreased stress and anxiety and improved mood and concentration. Furthermore, plyometrics and callisthenics are practical anaerobic activities that can be done safely at home or in a specialised training environment (Mikkelsen et al., 2017; Vancampfort et al., 2017).

Despite the evidence for plyometrics' benefits and callisthenics' treatment of PTSD, Knapik et al. (2003) suggest some potential drawbacks. First, plyometrics and callisthenics can be strenuous for individuals with

PTSD, as they may trigger flashbacks or other traumatic memories, such as memories of engagements with enemy gunfire (Begin et al., 2019). Moreover, it may be difficult for individuals with PTSD to adhere to a structured plyometrics and callisthenics routine due to low mood and lacking motivation or energy (Verstrael et al., 2013; Hegberg et al., 2019). Additionally, plyometrics and callisthenics may not be feasible for individuals with PTSD due to additional physical disabilities that limit their participation in plyometrics and callisthenics exercises (Rosenbaum et al., 2015).

Finally, the current research into plyometrics and callisthenics and PTSD is minimal and has limitations, such as small sample sizes, leading to mixed findings (Knapik et al., 2003; Michailidis et al., 2013). Therefore, more detailed research into the potential benefits of plyometrics and callisthenics is required to assess its suitability in providing a possible treatment option for veterans with PTSD.

Flexibility Exercise

Stretching, another name for flexibility exercises, is a physical activity that tries to increase the range of motion in the body's joints and muscles (Dick et al., 2014). In addition, Proprioceptive Neuromuscular Facilitation (PNF) stretching, dynamic stretching, and static stretching are a few of the different ways that flexibility exercises can be carried out (Frederick & Frederick, 2020). Moreover, flexibility exercises or stretching is often performed as part of a warm-up before, during the cool-down after a workout, or as an activity on their own (Frederick & Frederick, 2020). Furthermore, flexibility exercises can be done in various settings, including at home, in a gym, or outdoors (Dick et al., 2014).

Static stretching is a flexibility exercise that involves holding a stretch in place for a prolonged period of time; dynamic stretching requires moving the muscles through a range of motion. In addition, static and dynamic stretching and tightening and relaxing the muscles are all components of PNF stretching, which aims to promote flexibility (Frederick & Frederick, 2020). Moreover, Dick et al. (2014) suggest flexibility exercises increase the range of motion in the joints and improve strength, balance, and mindfulness.

According to Huberty et al. (2020), flexibility exercise is recommended for people of all ages and fitness levels, and it is a crucial part of living a healthy lifestyle. Moreover, for adults to maintain optimal cardiovascular health, the World Health Organization (WHO) recommends engaging in at least 150 minutes of moderate exercise or 75 minutes of vigorous-intensity exercise per week (Patel et al., 2017). Furthermore, to maintain a balanced training routine, it is recommended to engage in at least two flexibility exercise sessions in addition to regular aerobic exercise training (Huberty et al., 2020).

Physiological Benefits of Flexibility Exercise

Flexibility exercise has a range of physiological effects on the body, with stretching supporting the flexibility and range of motion of the body's joints and muscles (Groer et al., 2015). In addition, routine stretching aids muscle fibre recruitment and helps to improve physical performance and reduces injury (Roy-Byrne et al., 2008). Moreover, Dick et al. (2014) found that individuals who engaged in stretching increased blood flow and oxygen delivery to the muscles, which improved concentration and reduced anxiety (Frederick & Frederick, 2020).

In addition, flexibility exercises such as stretching, yoga and Pilates are good for improving muscular strength, power, and endurance (Groer et al., 2015). Likewise, flexibility exercise promotes lowering body fat, and building muscle and can enhance body composition and general health. Additionally, regular flexibility exercise can promote relaxation in individuals with PTSD, and reduce stress and anxiety (Roy-Byrne et al., 2008; Sato et al., 2003).

Finally, flexibility exercise can positively affect the brain and mental health (Andrews & Jenkins, 2019; Heath & Beattie, 2019). Moreover, Cole et al. (2022) found flexibility exercise to enhance cognitive abilities such as memory, attention, and processing speed. Additionally, participation in flexibility exercise increases the body's natural feel-good chemicals, endorphins, which can elevate mood and lessen the signs of sadness and anxiety (Cole et al., 2022).

Flexibility Exercise as a PTSD Treatment

Research into flexibility exercise is not as extensive as aerobic or anaerobic exercise. However, flexibility exercise has been identified as a viable alternative therapy for mental health, including anxiety, depression, and PTSD (Albright & Thyer, 2010; Dick et al., 2014). Moreover, flexibility exercise has provided some benefits in treating PTSD because it promotes relaxation, and improves sleep quality, as well as lowering agitation and depressive symptoms (Capon et al., 2019). Additionally, Smith and Merwin

(2021) point to the release of endorphins during flexibility exercise being a significant contribution to supporting the treatment of complex PTSD symptoms, such as avoidance behaviours and negative thoughts. Furthermore, deep breathing, progressive muscle relaxation, meditation, and yoga have been shown to produce endorphins, neurotransmitters naturally produced by the brain, that have anti-anxiety and anti-pain properties (Martland et al., 2020; Smith & Merwin, 2021).

In addition, Asmundson et al. (2013) suggest the endorphins released during relaxation and flexibility exercise aid in decreasing symptoms of stress, anxiety, and depression commonly associated with PTSD. Moreover, bouts of flexibility exercise have been shown to reduce anger, anxiety, and social avoidance (Asmundson et al., 2013).

According to Cole et al. (2022), flexibility exercises such as yoga and Pilates can help ease PTSD symptoms. In addition, these exercises are accessible to many people and adaptable to abilities and fitness goals and are simple to include in daily activities (Heath & Beattie, 2019). Moreover, research has revealed that flexibility exercises have been found to improve mood and relieve stress (Lopes-Silva et al., 2018). Furthermore, flexibility exercises led to decreased symptoms of anxiety and depression and enhanced sleep among individuals with PTSD (Frederick & Frederick, 2020). Therefore, this section will cover the relationship between flexibility exercises and PTSD symptomology.

Flexibility Exercise and PTSD Symptomology

Pilates and Yoga

Pilates and yoga, recognised as forms of flexibility exercises, are frequently utilised to enhance strength, power, and agility, as noted by Michailidis et al. (2013). Moreover, Ratamess (2021) emphasises in his recent Chapter that plyometrics constitutes an intense physical activity involving rapid and forceful movements, aiming to amplify power, speed, and agility. Furthermore, Breitbach et al. conducted research demonstrating that calisthenics exercises rely exclusively on the body's own weight as resistance, promoting improvements in strength, endurance, and flexibility. Additionally, Pilates and yoga have gained significant popularity for their potential to enhance physical performance and alleviate symptoms of anxiety, as observed by Groer et al. (2015) and Hegberg et al. (2019).

In addition, Pilates and yoga are extremely popular as a form of flexibility exercise, and are utilised to improve agility, strength, power, and cardiovascular health, which has led to improved sleep quality (Groer et al., 2015; Taylor et al., 2020). Moreover, Breitbach et al. found Pilates and yoga to involve a combination of aerobic and strength training to improve cardiovascular fitness and overall well-being, which has led to decreased stress and anxiety and improved mood and concentration. Furthermore, Pilates and yoga are practical flexibility exercises that can be done safely at home or in a specialised training environment (Knowles et al., 2019; Huberty et al., 2020).

Despite the evidence for the benefits of Pilates and yoga in treating PTSD, Lang et al. (2021) suggest some potential drawbacks. First, Pilates and yoga can be strenuous for individuals with PTSD, as they may trigger flashbacks or other traumatic memories, such as engagements with enemy gunfire (Begin et al., 2019). Moreover, it may be difficult for individuals with PTSD to adhere to a structured Pilates and yoga routine due to low mood and lacking energy (Allen et al., 2018; Hegberg et al., 2019). Additionally, Pilates and yoga may not be feasible for individuals with PTSD due to additional physical disabilities that limit their participation (Groer et al., 2015). Finally, the current research into Pilates, yoga and PTSD has minimal limitations, such as small sample sizes, which have led to mixed findings (Lang et al., 2021). Therefore, more detailed research into the potential benefits of Pilates and yoga is required to assess their suitability in providing a possible treatment option for veterans with PTSD.

Functional Types of Physical Exercise

Functional exercise is a physical activity that enhances a person's capacity to carry out everyday tasks and movements, such as walking, lifting, and bending (Izquierdo et al., 2021). In addition, functional exercise stresses the whole body, recruiting motions that imitate real-life activities, unlike traditional exercise, which may target muscle groups or body regions (Martland et al., 2020). Moreover, functional exercise includes balance, mind-body, High-Intensity Interval Training (HIIT), and CrossFit (Claudino et al., 2018; Izquierdo et al., 2021).

Functional exercise is intended to increase general fitness and improve a person's capacity to carry out tasks of daily living, including moving heavy objects or ascending stairs, more effectively, and efficiently. Moreover, functional exercise usually entails a combination of flexibility, strength, and endurance training that can be tailored to the goals and skills of people at every fitness level (Heywood, 2015). This section will examine the physiological effects of functional exercise and its applicability as a therapy for PTSD treatment in veterans.

Physiological Impacts of Functional Types of Exercise

Functional exercise has been demonstrated to help people with PTSD physiologically and psychologically (Wildgoose, 2019). For example, functional exercise may benefit PTSD patients physiologically by improving cardiovascular health, reducing blood pressure and body fat percentage, and building more robust, resilient muscles (Brewin et al., 2012; Plag et al., 2020). In addition, functional exercise can help improve sleep, which is advantageous for people with PTSD, who typically struggle with sleep issues (Plag et al., 2020).

Functional exercise is a form of therapy that has been shown to have psychological benefits for individuals with PTSD (Ashdown-Franks et al., 2019; Bozdarov et al., 2022). Additionally, Hegberg et al. (2019) suggest that functional exercise may aid in treating PTSD through both aerobic and anaerobic mechanisms. Such exercises can also help individuals with PTSD regain control over their bodies and enhance their self-esteem (Bozdarov et al., 2022).

Functional exercise has been found to impact several neurological pathways, including exposure to and desensitisation to internal arousal cues, enhanced cognitive function, exercise-induced neuroplasticity, and normalisation of inflammatory and HPA markers, as described by Hegberg et al. (2019). Regularly incorporating functional exercise into one's lifestyle can result in numerous physiological and psychological benefits that improve overall health and well-being. In this section, we will explore recent research on specialised functional exercise and its potential therapeutic use in managing PTSD.

Functional Types of Exercise as a PTSD Treatment

Tai chi, qigong, dance, High-Intensity Interval Training (HIIT) and CrossFit are all forms of functional exercise that are designed to prioritise the development of stability and balance (Papazoglou & Andersen, 2014; Steinberg-Oren et al., 2016). In addition, Steinberg-Oren et al. (2016) suggest that low-impact dance and movement Programmes have provided veterans with an alternative approach to treating PTSD (Zhu et al., 2022).

Furthermore, exercises replicating real-world movements and actions, including farmers' carries, box hops, stair climbs, tyre flipping, and rope climbing, have successfully enhanced physical health and aided recovery from PTSD, reducing anxiety, depression, and stress cues by working on mental toughness (Heywood, 2015; Petz, 2021).

Functional exercises, such as Tai chi, qigong, dance, High-Intensity Interval Training (HIIT), and CrossFit, have also been identified by Papazoglou and Andersen (2014) as potential therapeutic tools to ease PTSD symptoms. Furthermore, these exercises are adaptable to various fitness goals and abilities, making them accessible to a broad range of individuals (Ferrer & Davis, 2019). Moreover, research has revealed that the feeling of community associated with functional movement exercises can improve mood and reduce stress (Gogojewicz et al., 2020). Furthermore, functional movement exercises decrease anxiety and avoidance symptoms, which leads to improved sleep quality in individuals with PTSD (Martland et al., 2020; Plag et al., 2020). Therefore, this section will cover the relationship between flexibility exercises, specifically HITT and CrossFit and PTSD symptomology.

High-Intensity Interval Training (HIIT)

High-Intensity Interval Training (HIIT) is a form of functional exercise and consists of performing short bursts of intense anaerobic exercise, followed by extended recovery periods, and is designed to push the body to its physical limits (Martland et al., 2020; Plag et al., 2020). In addition, HIIT workouts are effective in improving cardiovascular fitness and building endurance, while burning fat and can lower levels of anxiety and depression and improve self-esteem (Martland et al., 2020). Similarly, individuals with PTSD who engage in HIIT have improved sleep and self-esteem (Patel et al., 2017). Furthermore, this form of functional exercise is intense, challenging, and demanding employing the core, lower and upper body muscles to maintain balance and stability (Martland et al., 2020; Plag et al., 2020).

HIIT is growing in popularity as a form of functional movement exercise in the veteran community, and is utilised to improve stamina and strength, which has led to improved sleep quality (Mobbs & Bonanno, 2018). Moreover, Mobbs and Bonanno (2018) found HIIT requires increased muscle activation and increases in energy expenditure, leading to improved self-confidence and a decrease in anxiety and depression.

Furthermore, HIIT is an effective anaerobic activity that can improve overall health and fitness and can be done safely at home or in a specialised training environment (Mobbs & Bonanno, 2018; Plag et al., 2020). Moreover, Whitworth et al. (2019) found that HIIT has many advantages for helping PTSD-affected veterans manage fight, flight, or freeze responses.

Despite the evidence for the benefits of HIIT in treating PTSD, Steinberg-Oren et al. (2016) suggest some potential drawbacks. First, HIIT can be extremely strenuous for individuals with PTSD, as it may trigger intrusive memories and traumatic flashbacks of battlefield experiences of gunbattles with the enemy and indirect fire explosions (Hall et al., 2020). Moreover, it may be difficult for individuals with PTSD to adhere to a structured HIIT training schedule due to low mood and lacking motivation or energy (Poon, 2022). Second, HIIT may not be feasible for individuals with PTSD due to additional physical disabilities that limit their participation (Engelhard et al., 2007). Finally, the current research into HIIT and PTSD is minimal and inconclusive, with several limitations, such as small sample sizes, which have led to mixed findings (Engelhard et al., 2007). Therefore, more detailed research into the potential benefits of HIIT is required to evaluate its suitability in providing a possible treatment option for veterans with PTSD.

CrossFit®

CrossFit® is a fitness regime that is performed using a variety of functional movement exercises and was invented by Greg Glassman in 2000, with the first CrossFit® gym, known as a "Box", opened in 2001 (Claudino et al., 2018). In addition, CrossFit® focuses on being competent in various physical attributes by performing a combination of physically demanding functional movement exercises, HIIT, and Olympic weightlifting techniques (Drake et al., 2017; Petz, 2021). Moreover, Ferrer and Davis (2019) found that by combining functional movements, significant adaptations with cardiovascular fitness, endurance, strength, power, speed and agility, balance, and flexibility are core pillars of CrossFit® sessions. Furthermore, nutrition, recovery, and mental toughness are equally vital components of CrossFit®, which encourages all who participate to prioritise a healthy and balanced diet while encouraging appropriate rest and recovery, at the same time as developing mental resilience (Claudino et al.,

2018; Petz, 2021). Finally, CrossFit® is a brand, and during my research, I sought and gained permission to use the CrossFit® Brand name.

CrossFit® is growing in popularity as a form of functional movement exercise in the veteran community, and it is being utilised to improve overall physical well-being, which has led to improved sleep and a reduction in avoidance behaviours (Claudino et al., 2018). Moreover, Petz (2021) found the community approach to exercise associated with CrossFit® has been recognised with improvements in self-confidence and a decrease in anxiety and depression. Furthermore, CrossFit® is an effective multi-functional high-intensity anaerobic activity that can be adjusted for individuals' fitness abilities, improving overall cardiovascular health. It can be done safely at home without equipment or a CrossFit® box (Claudino et al., 2018; Petz, 2021).

Poston et al. (2016) found that while there is some evidence supporting the use of CrossFit® in treating PTSD, there are also potential drawbacks, as highlighted by Klimek et al. (2018). CrossFit® can be highly strenuous for individuals with PTSD, potentially triggering traumatic memories and flashbacks. In addition, adhering to a structured HIIT training schedule may be challenging for those with PTSD due to low mood, lack of motivation or energy (Poon, 2022), and additional physical disabilities that limit participation (Drake et al., 2017). Moreover, the current research on HIIT and PTSD is limited and inconclusive, with several limitations, such as small sample sizes, leading to mixed findings. Therefore, it is necessary to conduct more detailed research to assess the suitability of HIIT as a potential treatment option for veterans with PTSD.

Chapter Conclusion

This chapter explored the various types of physical exercises to assess their suitability as potential treatments for military veterans with PTSD. Throughout this investigation, physical activity is used universally in society as a well-established pillar of cardiovascular fitness and overall well-being (McArdle et al., 2010; Patel et al., 2017). Additionally, Hegberg et al. (2019) point to physical exercise being found in many forms, including aerobic exercise, anaerobic activity, flexibility training, and functional exercise, each with unique benefits to physical and mental health (Papazoglou & Andersen, 2014; Hegberg et al., 2019).

In addition, the link between physical exercise and PTSD is mixed and complex, with each form of physical exercise providing various therapeutic benefits.

Aerobic exercises like walking, running, and swimming improve cardiovascular health and have been found to lessen PTSD symptoms, including anxiety and depression, diminish hyperarousal, and enhance sleep quality (Claudino et al., 2018; Hegberg et al., 2019; Petz, 2021).

Further, anaerobic exercises, such as weightlifting, resistance training and sprinting, improve muscle strength and power, decrease anger, avoidance behaviours, and emotional stress cues (Smith & Merwin, 2021). In addition, Michailidis et al. (2013) found flexibility exercises, such as Pilates, yoga and stretching, are crucial in easing muscle tension, promoting calmness, and reducing stress and anxiety symptoms. Furthermore, Mobbs and Bonanno (2018) found that functional exercises like Tai chi, qigong, dance, HIIT, and CrossFit® are successful in improving overall fitness and practical functioning, while also aiding improvements in self-confidence and decreasing anxiety, depression, and avoidance behaviours.

Despite the evidence for the benefits of physical exercise in treating PTSD, Hegberg et al. (2019) suggest some potential drawbacks. First, physical exercise can be highly strenuous for individuals with PTSD, as it may trigger traumatic memories and flashbacks (Klimek et al., 2018). Moreover, physical exercise may not be easily assessable for all veterans with PTSD, especially veterans with physical disabilities (Björkman & Ekblom, 2022). Furthermore, the findings from existing literature are conflicting, this may be due to small sample sizes and lack any long-term results, which limit any treatment recommendations, and there is a need for further research into physical exercise as a potential treatment for military veterans with PTSD (Abeyasinghe et al., 2012; Hegberg et al., 2019).

From the exploration of current PTSD treatment modalities to the investigation of physical exercise as a treatment modality marks the conclusion of the literature review. In the upcoming methodology chapter, we will shift our focus to outlining the framework for conducting new research.

References

Abeyasinghe, A. M., Baker, C., Charlton, R., & Smith, F. (2012). The importance of physical fitness for military personnel. *Journal of the Royal Army Medical Corps, 158*(2), 123–127.

Albright, D. L., & Thyer, B. A. (2010). Does exercise training alleviate depression in older adults? *Journal of Gerontological Social Work, 53*(4), 347–357.

Allen, A. P., Kennedy, P. J., Cryan, J. F., Dinan, T. G., & Clarke, G. (2018). Biological and psychological markers of stress in humans: Focus on the Trier Social Stress Test. *Neuroscience & Biobehavioral Reviews, 38*(1), 94–124.

American College of Sports Medicine. (2003). *ACSM fitness book* (3rd ed.). Human Kinetics.

Anderson, E., & Shivakumar, G. (2013). Effects of exercise and physical activity on anxiety. *Frontiers in Psychiatry, 4*, 27.

Andrewes, S. G., & Jenkins, L. (2019). Exercise as a therapeutic intervention for PTSD. *Mental Health and Physical Activity, 16*(1), 3–9.

Arem, H., Moore, S. C., Patel, A., Hartge, P., de Gonzalez, A. B., Visvanathan, K., et al. (2015). Leisure time physical activity and mortality: A detailed pooled analysis of the dose-response relationship. *JAMA Internal Medicine, 175*(6), 959–967.

Ashdown-Franks, G., Firth, J., Carney, R., Carvalho, A. F., Hallgren, M., Koyanagi, A., et al. (2019). Exercise as medicine for mental and substance use disorders: A meta-review of the benefits for neuropsychiatric and cognitive outcomes. *Sports Medicine, 50*(1), 151–170.

Asmundson, G. J. G., Fetzner, M. G., DeBoer, L. B., Powers, M. B., Otto, M. W., & Smits, J. A. J. (2013). Let's get physical: A contemporary review of the anxiolytic effects of exercise for anxiety and its disorders. *Depression and Anxiety, 30*(4), 362–373.

Babson, K. A., Heinz, A. J., & Bonn-Miller, M. O. (2015). Sleep, PTSD, and substance use: An update and clinical review. *Current Psychiatry Reports, 17*(3), 22.

Begin, M., Benoit, D., & Robitaille, M. (2019). Resistance training in trauma rehabilitation: A systematic review. *Military Medicine, 184*(5–6), e123–e131.

Bernard, P., Romain, A. J., Caudroit, J., Chevance, G., Carayol, M., Gourlan, M., et al. (2021). Exercise and PTSD: A systematic review and meta-analysis. *Psychiatry Research, 295*, 113629.

Bessman, S. P., & Carpenter, C. L. (1985). The creatine-creatine phosphate energy shuttle. *Annual Review of Biochemistry, 54*, 831–862.

Bestha, D. P., Krishnamurthy, N., & Chakraborty, S. (2018). Effect of aerobic exercise on mental health: A systematic review. *International Journal of Physiology, Nutrition and Physical Education, 3*(2), 985–989.

Bettmann, J. E., Mortensen, J. M., & Power, M. J. (2016). Wilderness therapy with adolescents: A systematic review. *Child and Adolescent Social Work Journal, 33*(6), 543–559.

Bettmann, J. E., Tucker, A., Behrens, E., & Vanderloo, M. (2021). Outdoor behavioral healthcare: A review of research. *Journal of Therapeutic Schools and Programs, 9*(1), 35–52.

Bichler, C. S., Skaar, N. R., & Hartwig, E. K. (2022). Walking as therapy: Exploring the impact on veterans with PTSD. *Journal of Military and Veterans Health, 30*(2), 12–19.

Björkman, A., & Ekblom, M. M. (2022). Exercise and stress resilience in veterans. *Scandinavian Journal of Medicine & Science in Sports, 32*(5), 820–830.

Bloomer, R. J., Goldfarb, A. H., Wideman, L., McKenzie, M. J., & Consitt, L. A. (2005). Effects of acute aerobic and anaerobic exercise on blood markers of oxidative stress. *Journal of Strength and Conditioning Research, 19*(2), 276–285.

Borghi-Silva, A., Mendes, R. G., Trimer, R., & Oliveira, C. R. (2009). Respiratory responses to aerobic training in COPD patients. *Respiratory Medicine, 103*(5), 730–738.

Bozdarov, J., Petrov, A., & Dimitrov, M. (2022). Functional training for veterans with PTSD: A randomized controlled trial. *Military Psychology, 34*(6), 421–432.

Brackley, C., Fox, R., & Richardson, J. (2020). Swimming as therapy: Mental health outcomes in veterans. *Therapeutic Advances in Psychopharmacology, 10*, 2045125320940112.

Bremner, J. D., & Marmar, C. R. (2002). Trauma, memory, and dissociation. In J. D. Bremner & C. R. Marmar (Eds.), *Trauma, memory, and dissociation* (pp. 1–22). American Psychiatric Press.

Brewin, C. R., Andrews, B., & Hejdenberg, J. (2012). Recognition and treatment of psychological disorders during military service in the UK armed forces: a study of war pensioners. *Social Psychiatry and Psychiatric Epidemiology, 47*(12), 1891–1897.

Brewin, C. R., Dalgleish, T., & Joseph, S. (2017). Reconsolidation in memory therapy: PTSD implications. *Psychological Medicine, 47*(14), 2486–2494.

Brewin, C. R., Garnett, R., & Andrews, B. (2011). Trauma, identity and mental health in UK veterans. *Journal of Traumatic Stress, 24*(5), 682–689.

Brewin, C. R., Gregory, J. D., Lipton, M., & Burgess, N. (2010). Intrusive images in psychological disorders: Characteristics, neural mechanisms, and treatment implications. *Psychological Review, 117*(1), 210–232.

Brittain, I., & Green, S. (2012). Disability sport is a vehicle for social inclusion: A critical review. *Disability & Society, 27*(7), 1107–1122.

Broman-Fulks, J. J., Berman, M. E., Rabian, B. A., & Webster, M. J. (2004). Effects of aerobic exercise on anxiety sensitivity. *Behaviour Research and Therapy, 42*(2), 125–136.

Bryan, M. A., et al. (2018). Hiking and mental health: A systematic review. *Ecopsychology, 10*(4), 196–204.

Burke, S. M., & Utley, A. (2013). Climbing towards recovery: Outdoor adventure for veterans. *Journal of Adventure Education and Outdoor Learning, 13*(1), 69–83.

Caddick, N., & Smith, B. (2014). The impact of sport and physical activity on the well-being of combat veterans: A systematic review. *Psychology of Sport and Exercise, 15*(1), 9–18.

Caddick, N., & Smith, B. (2018). Exercise as a catalyst for recovery stories: A narrative study of veterans living with PTSD. *Qualitative Health Research, 28*(3), 564–577.

Callaghan, P. (2004). Exercise: A neglected intervention in mental health care? *Journal of Psychiatric and Mental Health Nursing, 11*(4), 476–483.

Capon, H., Hallgren, M., & Stubbs, B. (2019). Yoga, mindfulness and PTSD: A systematic review. *Journal of Psychiatric Research, 113*, 174–182.

Carek, P. J., Laibstain, S. E., & Carek, S. M. (2011). Exercise for the treatment of depression and anxiety. *International Journal of Psychiatry in Medicine, 41*(1), 15–28.

Celano, C. M., Huffman, J. C., & Mastromauro, C. (2016). Depression and anxiety in cardiac patients: The role of exercise. *Current Cardiovascular Risk Reports, 10*(5), 12–20.

Claudi-no, J. G., Gabbett, T. J., Bourgeois, F., Souza, H. S., Miranda, R. C., Mezencio, B., et al. (2018). CrossFit®: Exercise characteristics and potential health benefits. *Sports Medicine, 48*(4), 787–801.

Cloitre, M. (2009). Effective psychotherapies for PTSD: A review and critique. *Journal of Clinical Psychology, 65*(8), 841–862.

Colcombe, S. J., Erickson, K. I., Scalf, P. E., Kim, J. S., Prakash, R., McAuley, E., et al. (2006). Aerobic exercise training increases brain volume in aging humans. *Journal of Gerontology: Medical Sciences, 61A*(11), 1166–1170.

Cole, S., Berman, J., & Huber, D. (2022). Aquatic therapies in PTSD: Outcomes and mechanisms. *Frontiers in Psychiatry, 13*, 789–799.

Collins, S., & Long, A. (2003). Working with the psychological effects of trauma: Consequences for mental health-care workers. *Journal of Psychiatric and Mental Health Nursing, 10*(4), 417–424.

Connell, R. (2016). *Masculinities* (2nd ed.). Polity Press.

Connell, R. W., & Messerschmidt, J. W. (2005). Hegemonic masculinity: Rethinking the concept. *Gender & Society, 19*(6), 829–859.

Cook, N. R. (2003). Statistical evaluation of interventions: Implications for clinical trials. *Statistics in Medicine, 22*(2), 313–321.

Cooper, R. A., & Quatrano, L. A. (1999). Research on physical activity and disability: An emerging national priority. *Medicine & Science in Sports & Exercise, 31*(10), S535–S541.

Cordier, R., Milbourn, B., Martin, R., Buchanan, A., Chung, D., & Speyer, R. (2019). The role of community-based exercise programs for veterans with PTSD. *Disability and Rehabilitation, 41*(19), 2294–2302.

Crombie, A. P., Leitzmann, M. F., & Troiano, R. P. (2019). Physical activity and public health: An evidence overview. *Public Health Reports, 134*(2), 136–142.

Crombie, A. P., Singh, A., & Roberts, C. K. (2023). Aerobic exercise in PTSD: Mechanisms and outcomes. *Exercise and Sport Sciences Reviews, 51*(1), 23–31.

Danto, E. (2016). *Historical research in the social work profession*. Columbia University Press.

Davidson, P. R., & Parker, K. C. H. (2001). Eye movement desensitization and reprocessing (EMDR): A meta-analysis. *Journal of Consulting and Clinical Psychology, 69*(2), 305–316.

Davis-Berman, J., Berman, D. S., & Capone, R. (2018). Therapeutic benefits of outdoor activities for trauma survivors. *Journal of Experiential Education, 41*(2), 123–140.

De Vries, J. D., van Hooff, M. L., & Geurts, S. A. (2012). Exercise to reduce work-related fatigue among employees: A randomized trial. *Scandinavian Journal of Work, Environment & Health, 38*(2), 120–133.

Diaz, A., & Motta, R. (2008). The effects of aerobic exercise on anxiety and depression among female college students. *College Student Journal, 42*(2), 630–642.

Dick, R., Agostinelli, G., & Nielsen, R. (2014). Stretching, flexibility, and mental health outcomes: A clinical review. *International Journal of Therapy and Rehabilitation, 21*(9), 432–440.

Drake, D., Feller, S., & Craig, A. (2017). CrossFit® and veterans: Exploring clinical impacts. *Journal of Military Medicine, 182*(1–2), e1900–e1906.

Eckstrom, E., Voss, C., & Hsu, C. (2020). Swimming and rehabilitation outcomes in older adults. *Geriatrics, 75*(3), 305–314.

Ehlers, A., Clark, D. M., Hackmann, A., McManus, F., & Fennell, M. (2005). Cognitive therapy for PTSD: Development and evaluation. *Behaviour Research and Therapy, 43*(4), 413–431.

Elbogen, E. B., Johnson, S. C., Newton, V. M., Straits-Troster, K., Vasterling, J. J., Wagner, H. R., & Beckham, J. C. (2019). Criminal justice involvement and PTSD in military veterans. *Law and Human Behaviour, 43*(2), 99–110.

Engelhard, I. M., van den Hout, M. A., & McNally, R. J. (2007). Memory and posttraumatic stress disorder: The role of mental imagery. *Applied Cognitive Psychology, 21*(3), 387–403.

Feduccia, A. A., & Mithoefer, M. C. (2018). MDMA-assisted psychotherapy for PTSD: A review. *Journal of Psychopharmacology, 32*(7), 725–737.

Ferrer, D. A., & Davis, R. W. (2019). CrossFit and veterans' rehabilitation: A qualitative study. *Journal of Veterans Studies, 5*(2), 83–97.

Finley, E. P. (2011). *Fields of combat: Understanding PTSD among veterans of Iraq and Afghanistan*. Cornell University Press.

Foa, E. B., Keane, T. M., Friedman, M. J., & Cohen, J. A. (2018). *Effective treatments for PTSD: Practice guidelines from the International Society for Traumatic Stress Studies* (3rd ed.). Guilford Press.

Folkins, C. H., & Sime, W. E. (1981). Physical fitness training and mental health. *American Psychologist, 36*(4), 373–389.

Foote, C. E., Szabo, A. N., & Roper, L. (2015). Aquatic exercise interventions for PTSD. *Journal of Aquatic Therapy, 23*(4), 12–20.

Frederick, A., & Frederick, C. (2020). Stretching and mental health: Evidence from clinical practice. *Complementary Therapies in Medicine, 51*, 102414.

Frontera, W. R., Dawson, D. M., & Slovik, D. M. (2006). *Exercise physiology: Human performance and clinical applications* (2nd ed.). Human Kinetics.

Gates, N., Valenzuela, M., Sachdev, P. S., & Singh, M. F. (2012). Psychological wellbeing and aerobic exercise: A review. *Sports Medicine, 42*(5), 367–376.

Gogojewicz, A., Tafil-Klawe, M., & Nowak, Z. (2020). Functional training and psychological resilience in PTSD. *Journal of Strength and Conditioning Research, 34*(3), 789–796.

Goldstein, E., Topitzes, J., & Mersky, J. P. (2018). Cycling as an intervention for trauma recovery: Evidence and applications. *Journal of Clinical Sport Psychology, 12*(4), 650–664.

Greist, J. H., Klein, M. H., Eischens, R. R., Faris, J., Gurman, A. S., & Morgan, W. P. (1979). Running as treatment for depression. *Comprehensive Psychiatry, 20*(1), 41–54.

Groer, M. W., Kane, B., & Williams, S. (2015). Exercise, immunity, and PTSD. *Journal of Psychosomatic Research, 78*(6), 578–585.

Hall, K. S., Morey, M. C., & Bosworth, H. B. (2016). Veterans' exercise patterns: Associations with health outcomes. *Preventive Medicine, 88*, 188–194.

Hall, K. S., Sloane, R., & Pieper, C. F. (2020). Exercise and PTSD: A systematic review of veteran interventions. *American Journal of Lifestyle Medicine, 14*(2), 123–135.

Hall, L., & Knuth, S. (2019). Walking programs for veterans: Mental health and social outcomes. *Journal of Rehabilitation Research and Development, 56*(3), 415–423.

Heath, C., & Beattie, S. (2019). Yoga and mental health in trauma survivors. *International Journal of Yoga Therapy, 29*(1), 45–53.

Hegberg, N. J., Hayes, J. P., & Hayes, S. M. (2019). Exercise intervention in PTSD: A narrative review and rationale for implementation. *Frontiers in Psychiatry, 10*, 133.

Heywood, V. (2015). Functional fitness for clinical populations. *Journal of Clinical Exercise Physiology, 4*(2), 10–19.

Hoge, C. W., Auchterlonie, J. L., & Milliken, C. S. (2007). Mental health problems, use of mental health services, and attrition from military service after Iraq war deployment. *New England Journal of Medicine, 357*(6), 453–463.

Huberty, J. L., Green, J., & Puzia, M. (2020). Yoga and meditation in PTSD: Review of clinical trials. *Complementary Therapies in Clinical Practice, 39*, 101150.

Hupin, D., Roche, F., Gremeaux, V., Chatard, J. C., Oriol, M., Gaspoz, J. M., et al. (2015). Even a little physical activity is better for cardiovascular health. *European Journal of Preventive Cardiology, 22*(1), 23–29.

Izquierdo, M., Merchant, R. A., Morley, J. E., Anker, S. D., Aprahamian, I., Arai, H., et al. (2021). International exercise recommendations in older adults for prevention of frailty and falls: Consensus statement. *Age and Ageing, 50*(2), 1499–1509.

Jee, Y. (2016). Exercise and immunity. *Korean Journal of Pediatrics, 59*(9), 346–351.

Jones, T. A., Mueller, A., & Morris, S. (2020). Neuroplasticity and exercise interventions in PTSD. *Frontiers in Behavioural Neuroscience, 14*, 22.

Karlin, B. E., Ruzek, J. I., Chard, K. M., Eftekhari, A., Monson, C. M., Hembree, E. A., et al. (2010). Dissemination of evidence-based psychological treatments for posttraumatic stress disorder in the Veterans Health Administration. *Journal of Traumatic Stress, 23*(6), 663–673.

Kashihara, K., Maruyama, T., Murota, M., & Nakahara, Y. (2009). Positive effects of acute and moderate physical exercise on cognitive function. *Journal of Physiological Anthropology, 28*(4), 155–164.

Kirthika, P., Arulappan, J., & AlAmodi, A. A. (2019). Jump rope exercise and its psychological benefits in trauma-exposed individuals. *Journal of Clinical Sport Psychology, 13*(4), 585–598.

Klimek, L., Bergmann, K. C., Biedermann, T., Bousquet, J., Hellings, P. W., Jarvis, D., et al. (2018). Resistance training and immunological outcomes: Clinical implications. *Allergy, 73*(2), 242–252.

Knapik, J. J., Sharp, M. A., Canham-Chervak, M., Hauret, K., Patton, J. F., & Jones, B. H. (2003). Injury incidence and risk factors in military physical training. *Medicine & Science in Sports & Exercise, 35*(8), 1258–1266.

Knowles, R., Chadderton, H., & Cheston, R. (2019). Exercise groups for older veterans: Social support and mental health outcomes. *Aging & Mental Health, 23*(12), 1626–1634.

Kopacz, M. S., McCarten, J. M., Vance, C. G., & Connery, A. L. (2016). Exercise and chaplaincy: Opportunities for collaboration in veteran care. *Journal of Health Care Chaplaincy, 22*(4), 151–162.

Kraemer, W. J., Fleck, S. J., & Deschenes, M. R. (2002). *Exercise physiology: Integrating theory and application.* Lippincott Williams & Wilkins.

Kraemer, W. J., Ratamess, N. A., & French, D. N. (2004). Resistance training for health and performance. *Current Sports Medicine Reports, 3*(3), 165–171.

Lackey, Q., McKune, A., & Morris, C. (2021). Outdoor exercise and PTSD: Hiking interventions for military veterans. *Military Medicine, 186*(1–2), e182–e189.

Lang, A. J., Malaktaris, A. L., Casmar, P. V., & Jack, H. E. (2021). Yoga for veterans with PTSD: A systematic review and meta-analysis. *Journal of Alternative and Complementary Medicine, 27*(2), 83–95.

LeBouthillier, D. M., & Asmundson, G. J. G. (2017). The efficacy of resistance exercise in reducing anxiety sensitivity. *Journal of Anxiety Disorders, 47*, 87–96.

Leeb, S. (2018). The healing power of exercise: How movement impacts trauma recovery. *Journal of Holistic Nursing, 36*(2), 159–170.

Legarreta, M., Brown, J., & Smith, N. (2015). Exercise adherence in veterans with PTSD: Barriers and facilitators. *Occupational Therapy in Mental Health, 31*(4), 350–364.

Levine, P. A. (1997). *Waking the tiger: Healing trauma*. North Atlantic Books.

Levine, P. A. (2010). *In an unspoken voice: How the body releases trauma and restores goodness*. North Atlantic Books.

Ley, C., Barrio, M. R., Leach, L., & Bassett, S. (2018). Exercise interventions for people with PTSD in low-resource settings: A systematic review. *Psychology of Sport and Exercise, 38*, 61–71.

Lloret, S. P., Martinez, M., & Alvarez, J. (2021). Aquatic exercise and trauma recovery: Evidence from clinical populations. *Clinical Rehabilitation, 35*(10), 1423–1433.

Lopes-Silva, J. P., Silva, W. M., & Cesar, D. P. (2018). Energy systems contributions in high-intensity exercise. *Sports Medicine, 48*(4), 765–777.

Lucibello, K. M., Pigeon, W. R., & Bishop, T. M. (2020). Sleep, exercise, and PTSD: Clinical connections. *Sleep Medicine Clinics, 15*(1), 59–68.

Ma, S., Lee, Y., & Kim, H. (2021). Cycling and mental health: A review of benefits for trauma survivors. *Journal of Affective Disorders, 283*, 240–248.

Manger, T. A., & Motta, R. (2005). The impact of exercise on combat-related PTSD. *Military Psychology, 17*(1), 55–62.

Markotić, V., Mikulic, P., & Bratkovic, T. (2020). Physical activity and PTSD: A systematic review. *Croatian Medical Journal, 61*(2), 109–118.

Martland, R., Mondelli, V., & Stubbs, B. (2020). Exercise for the treatment of PTSD: A systematic review and meta-analysis. *Psychiatry Research, 284*, 112702.

Mazzardo-Martins, L., Martins, D. F., & Santos, A. R. (2010). Endorphin release during high-intensity exercise: Implications for trauma recovery. *Neuroscience Letters, 485*(1), 56–60.

McArdle, W. D., Katch, F. I., & Katch, V. L. (2010). *Exercise physiology: Nutrition, energy, and human performance* (7th ed.). Lippincott Williams & Wilkins.

McWeeny, S., O'Connor, R., & Patel, K. (2020). Military fitness training and PTSD rehabilitation. *Journal of Military Medicine, 185*(5–6), e715–e722.

Michailidis, Y., Fatouros, I. G., & Jamurtas, A. Z. (2013). Plyometric training, muscle damage and inflammation. *Sports Medicine, 43*(11), 997–1005.

Mikkelsen, K., Stojanovska, L., Polenakovic, M., Bosevski, M., & Apostolopoulos, V. (2017). Exercise and mental health. *Maturitas, 106*, 48–56.

Minton, K., Ogden, P., Pain, C., & Fisher, J. (2006). Somatic approaches to trauma therapy. *Journal of Bodywork and Movement Therapies, 10*(1), 1–9.

Mobbs, D., & Bonanno, G. A. (2018). Beyond resilience: Defining recovery from PTSD. *Clinical Psychology Review, 62*, 1–11.

Monson, C. M., Taft, C. T., & Fredman, S. J. (2009). Military-related PTSD and couple/family therapy. *Journal of Clinical Psychology, 65*(8), 711–724.

Murphy, D., Ashwick, R., Palmer, E., & Busuttil, W. (2016). Describing the profile of a population of UK veterans seeking support for PTSD. *European Journal of Psychotraumatology, 7*(1), 297–311.

Najavits, L. M. (2002). *Seeking safety: A treatment manual for PTSD and substance abuse*. Guilford Press.

Nanclerio, A., Russo, R., & Bianchi, G. (2022). Exercise programs in PTSD: Adherence and outcomes. *Journal of Psychiatric Research, 150*, 289–297.

Nisenbaum, R., Barrett, D. H., Reyes, M., Reeves, W. C., & Reeves, W. C. (2000). Deployment stressors and a chronic multisymptom illness among Gulf War veterans. *Journal of Nervous and Mental Disease, 188*(5), 259–266.

Nowacka-Chmielewska, M., Grabowski, J., & Wilczyńska, D. (2022). Neuroplasticity and PTSD: The role of exercise. *Progress in Neuro-Psychopharmacology & Biological Psychiatry, 112*, 110–118.

O'Donovan, G., Blazevich, A. J., Boreham, C., Cooper, A. R., Crank, H., Ekelund, U., et al. (2010). The ABC of physical activity for health: A consensus statement from the British Association of Sport and Exercise Sciences. *Journal of Sports Sciences, 28*(6), 573–591.

Oppizzi, L. M., & Umberger, R. (2018). Exercise interventions for PTSD: A review of clinical evidence. *Journal of Clinical Exercise Physiology, 7*(3), 43–50.

Otto, M. W., & Smits, J. A. J. (2011). *Exercise for mood and anxiety disorders: Translating science to practice*. Oxford University Press.

Owens, G. P., Baker, D. G., Kasckow, J., Ciesla, J. A., Mohamed, S., & Mohamed, S. (2012). Exercise and coping in veterans with PTSD. *Journal of Rehabilitation Research and Development, 49*(5), 775–784.

Paolucci, E. M., Loukov, D., Bowdish, D. M. E., & Heisz, J. J. (2018). Exercise reduces depression and inflammation but intensity matters. *Biological Psychology, 133*, 79–84.

Papazoglou, K., & Andersen, J. P. (2014). Yoga and mindfulness in first responders: Implications for PTSD. *Journal of Emergency Mental Health and Human Resilience, 16*(2), 110–112.

Patel, H., Alkhawam, H., Madanieh, R., Shah, N., Kosmas, C. E., & Vittorio, T. J. (2017). Aerobic vs anaerobic exercise training effects on the cardiovascular system. *World Journal of Cardiology, 9*(2), 134–144.

Patki, G., Solanki, N., Atrooz, F., Allam, F., Salim, S., & Salim, S. (2014). Novel role of aerobic exercise in modulating stress responses in PTSD. *Neuroscience Letters, 565*, 167–172.

Payne, P., Levine, P. A., & Crane-Godreau, M. A. (2015). Somatic experiencing: Using interoception and proprioception as core elements of trauma therapy. *Frontiers in Psychology, 6*, 93.

Pebole, M. M., & Hall, K. S. (2019). Physical activity interventions for PTSD: Mechanisms and outcomes. *Psychology of Sport and Exercise, 45*, 101–110.

Pebole, M. M., Hall, K. S., & Sliwinski, M. J. (2022). Jump rope exercise and PTSD: Pilot findings. *Mental Health and Physical Activity, 22*, 100439.

Pedersen, B. K., Saltin, B., & Zierath, J. R. (2017). Exercise as medicine: Evidence for prescribing exercise in chronic disease. *Scandinavian Journal of Medicine & Science in Sports, 27*(3), 32–38.

Petz, M. R. (2021). *CrossFit and functional training in PTSD rehabilitation*. Springer.

Plag, J., Ehlers, A., & Berger, W. (2020). HIIT in PTSD: A randomized controlled trial. *Journal of Affective Disorders, 276*, 572–579.

Plowman, S. A., & Smith, D. L. (2013). *Exercise physiology for health, fitness, and performance* (4th ed.). Lippincott Williams & Wilkins.

Poole, D. C., Burnley, M., Vanhatalo, A., Rossiter, H. B., & Jones, A. M. (2021). Critical power: An important fatigue threshold in exercise physiology. *Medicine & Science in Sports & Exercise, 53*(1), 194–206.

Poon, C. (2022). Adherence barriers in high-intensity exercise for trauma survivors. *Traumatology, 28*(2), 154–163.

Popovic, D., Simic, D., & Jovanovic, M. (2022). Exercise, stress regulation and PTSD: Current findings. *Psychiatry Research, 309*, 114–123.

Poston, W. S. C., Haddock, C. K., & Jahnke, S. A. (2016). Weightlifting, firefighting, and PTSD symptoms: A clinical study. *Journal of Occupational Health Psychology, 21*(2), 153–162.

Price, M., Gros, D. F., McCauley, J. L., Gros, K. S., Ruggiero, K. J., & Acierno, R. (2015). The role of physical activity in PTSD treatment: A randomized controlled trial. *Behaviour Research and Therapy, 62*, 33–41.

Qureshi, M., Pyne, J. M., Magruder, K. M., Schulz, P. E., & Kunik, M. E. (2011). The link between PTSD and physical health: Evidence from veteran populations. *General Hospital Psychiatry, 33*(2), 140–147.

Ratamess, N. A. (2021). *ACSM's foundations of strength training and conditioning*. Wolters Kluwer.

Rosenbaum, S., Vancampfort, D., Steel, Z., Newby, J., Ward, P. B., & Stubbs, B. (2015). Physical activity in the treatment of PTSD: A systematic review and meta-analysis. *Psychiatry Research, 230*(2), 130–136.

Rosenberger, M. E., Fulton, J. E., Buman, M. P., Troiano, R. P., Grandner, M. A., Buchner, D. M., et al. (2019). The 24-hour activity cycle: A new paradigm for physical activity. *Medicine & Science in Sports & Exercise, 51*(3), 454–464.

Ross, C. A., Dorahy, M. J., & Read, J. (2018). Dissociation and physical exercise in trauma survivors. *Journal of Trauma & Dissociation, 19*(4), 383–400.

Roy, T., Lloyd, C. E., Pouwer, F., Holt, R. I. G., & Snoek, F. J. (2010). Physical activity and glycaemic control in people with type 2 diabetes. *Diabetic Medicine, 27*(9), 1019–1027.

Roy-Byrne, P. P., Berliner, L., Zatzick, D., & Russo, J. (2008). Clinical management of PTSD. *BMJ, 336*(7652), 872–876.

Sadeghi, H., Moradi, N., & Haghshenas, A. (2022). Cycling and its psychological benefits in trauma recovery. *Journal of Rehabilitation Sciences, 18*(3), 220–228.

Sato, Y., Iwamoto, J., Kanoko, T., & Satoh, K. (2003). Low-intensity resistance training for elderly patients with osteoporosis. *American Journal of Medicine, 114*(4), 354–355.

Sawka, M. N. (2011). Physiology of exercise in military environments. In B. C. Nindl & S. J. Montain (Eds.), *Military performance physiology: Preparing soldiers for war* (pp. 53–74). CRC Press.

Schöner, J., Heinz, A., & Endres, M. (2017). Stress hormones and trauma recovery: The role of exercise. *Current Opinion in Psychiatry, 30*(3), 188–194.

Schuman, D. (2016). Veterans' narratives of mindfulness and exercise in trauma recovery. *Journal of Humanistic Psychology, 56*(2), 167–184.

Service, K. (2009). *Post-traumatic stress disorder: The essential guide.* Need2Know Books.

Shamus, E., & Cohen, S. (2009). Depressive symptom changes in patients receiving exercise interventions. *International Journal of Rehabilitation Research, 32*(1), 69–76.

Sharif, K., Watad, A., Bragazzi, N. L., Lichtbroun, M., Amital, H., & Shoenfeld, Y. (2018). Physical activity and autoimmune diseases: Get moving and manage the disease. *Autoimmunity Reviews, 17*(1), 53–72.

Shields, D., Kuhl, D., & Westwood, M. (2017). Moral injury, PTSD, and exercise in veterans. *Canadian Journal of Counselling and Psychotherapy, 51*(3), 175–190.

Singh, R., Khanna, R., & Jain, M. (2018). Exercise therapy for trauma survivors: An Indian perspective. *Indian Journal of Psychiatry, 60*(4), 503–509.

Smith, A. J., & Merwin, R. M. (2021). Exercise and acceptance-based interventions for PTSD. *Journal of Contextual Behavioural Science, 20*, 137–145.

Smith, P. J., Blumenthal, J. A., Hoffman, B. M., Cooper, H., Strauman, T. A., Welsh-Bohmer, K., et al. (2017). Aerobic exercise and neurocognitive performance: A meta-analytic review. *Psychosomatic Medicine, 72*(3), 239–252.

Speer, K., Semple, S., Naumovski, N., D'Cunha, N. M., McKune, A. J., & Georgousopoulou, E. N. (2019). Exercise interventions for PTSD: Biological mechanisms. *Neuroscience & Biobehavioural Reviews, 107*, 179–195.

Spurway, N. C. (1992). Aerobic and anaerobic pathways of energy supply during exercise. *British Medical Bulletin, 48*(3), 569–591.

Stallman, R. K. (2017). Swimming and mental health: From recreation to rehabilitation. *International Journal of Aquatic Research and Education, 11*(3), 1–14.

Stathopoulou, G., Powers, M. B., Berry, A. C., Smits, J. A., & Otto, M. W. (2006). Exercise interventions for mental health: A quantitative and qualitative review. *Clinical Psychology: Science and Practice, 13*(2), 179–193.

Steinberg-Oren, N., Regev, D., & Guez, J. (2016). Dance movement therapy for trauma survivors. *The Arts in Psychotherapy, 47*, 16–24.

Stern, A. F., Holder, N., & O'Connor, C. (2013). Adherence challenges in exercise interventions for PTSD. *European Journal of Psychotraumatology, 4*(1), 1–9.

Ströhle, A. (2007). Physical activity, exercise, depression and anxiety disorders. *Journal of Neural Transmission, 114*(9), 1253–1260.

Ströhle, A. (2019). Sports psychiatry: Mental health and performance in elite athletes. *European Archives of Psychiatry and Clinical Neuroscience, 269*(1), 1–3.

Stubbs, B., Vancampfort, D., Rosenbaum, S., Ward, P. B., Richards, J., Soundy, A., et al. (2017). Dropout rates in exercise interventions for adults with PTSD. *Journal of Psychiatric Research, 95*, 134–143.

Taylor, V., Garland, S. N., Kruse, S., & Carlson, L. E. (2020). Yoga for PTSD: A systematic review of the literature. *International Journal of Yoga Therapy, 30*(1), 49–58.

Tomlin, D. L., & Wenger, H. A. (2001). The relationship between aerobic fitness and recovery from high intensity intermittent exercise. *Sports Medicine, 31*(1), 1–11.

Tsukamoto, H., Suga, T., Takenaka, S., Tanaka, D., Takeuchi, T., Hamaoka, T., & Isaka, T. (2016). Repeated high-intensity interval exercise and its effect on oxygen uptake and endurance. *Journal of Applied Physiology, 121*(2), 563–572.

Van der Kolk, B. A. (1994). The body keeps the score: Memory and the evolving psychobiology of PTSD. *Harvard Review of Psychiatry, 1*(5), 253–265.

Van der Kolk, B. A. (2001). The psychobiology of PTSD. *Journal of Clinical Psychiatry, 62*(17), 16–24.

Van der Kolk, B. A. (2003). Posttraumatic stress disorder and the nature of trauma. *Dialogues in Clinical Neuroscience, 5*(3), 217–229.

Van der Kolk, B. A. (2006). Clinical implications of neuroscience research in PTSD. *Annals of the New York Academy of Sciences, 1071*(1), 277–293.

Van der Kolk, B. A. (2015). *The body keeps the score: Brain, mind, and body in the healing of trauma*. Viking.

Van der Kolk, B. A., Stone, L., West, J., Rhodes, A., Emerson, D., Suvak, M., & Spinazzola, J. (2014). Yoga as an adjunctive treatment for PTSD: A randomized controlled trial. *Journal of Clinical Psychiatry, 75*(6), e559–e565.

Van Gelderen, B. R., Nijdam, M. J., Haagen, J. F. G., & Vermetten, E. (2018). Meaning as a mechanism of change in PTSD treatment. *European Journal of Psychotraumatology, 9*(1), 1458577.

Vancampfort, D., Firth, J., Schuch, F. B., Rosenbaum, S., Mugisha, J., Hallgren, M., et al. (2017). Physical activity and sedentary behaviour in people with PTSD: A systematic review and meta-analysis. *Psychiatry Research, 256*, 102–114.

Varker, T., Brand, R. M., Ward, J., Terhaag, S., & Phelps, A. (2021). Efficacy of physical exercise in treating PTSD: A systematic review. *Journal of Anxiety Disorders, 80*, 102–113.

Verstrael, S., van der Heijden, P. G. M., & Sijbrandij, M. (2013). Exercise and PTSD treatment outcomes: A pilot study. *European Journal of Psychotraumatology, 4*(1), 1–8.

Wadley, G., & Le Rossignol, P. (1998). The relationship between repeated sprint ability and aerobic capacity. *Journal of Science and Medicine in Sport, 1*(2), 100–110.

Whitworth, J. W., & Ciccolo, J. T. (2016). Resistance training and PTSD: A review of literature. *Journal of Strength and Conditioning Research, 30*(12), 3501–3508.

Whitworth, J. W., Ciccolo, J. T., & Spalding, T. W. (2019). Exercise and PTSD in military veterans: A systematic review. *Military Medicine, 184*(9–10), e501–e508.

Wildgoose, K. (2019). Trauma-sensitive approaches to exercise and sport. *Journal of Sport Psychology in Action, 10*(2), 123–134.

Williamson, J. B., Heilman, K. M., & Heilman, K. M. (2013). Emotional regulation, exercise, and PTSD: Insights from neuropsychology. *Neuropsychology Review, 23*(4), 314–327.

Winett, R. A., & Ogletree, A. M. (2019). Evidence-based applications of exercise for mental health. *American Journal of Lifestyle Medicine, 13*(2), 155–165.

Wing, R. R., & Hill, J. O. (2001). Successful weight loss maintenance. *Annual Review of Nutrition, 21*(1), 323–341.

Zhu, M., Fang, Y., & Li, C. (2022). Dance interventions for PTSD: A systematic review and meta-analysis. *Frontiers in Psychology, 13*, 843218.

Zschucke, E., Gaudlitz, K., & Ströhle, A. (2013). Exercise and physical activity in mental disorders: Clinical and experimental evidence. *Journal of Preventive Medicine and Public Health, 46*(1), S12–S21.

Zupan, M. F., Arata, A. W., Dawson, L. H., Wile, A. L., Payn, T. L., & Hannon, M. E. (2009). Wingate anaerobic test peak power and anaerobic capacity classifications for men and women intercollegiate athletes. *Journal of Strength and Conditioning Research, 23*(9), 2598–2604.

CHAPTER 4

Reclaiming Myself Through CrossFit®: An Autoethnographic Analysis Informed by Self-Determination Theory

Each morning, I wake to echoes of combat, flashbacks that merge anger with fear and leave me adrift in regret and shame. Such intrusive memories typify Post-Traumatic Stress Disorder (PTSD) and erode both well-being and identity among military veterans (Able & Benedek, 2019). Conventional treatments can help, yet dropout, residual symptoms, and access barriers remain common. These limitations prompted me to search for complementary strategies to reclaim my life.

CrossFit® as a candidate intervention. After running, cycling, and weightlifting failed to ease my combat-related PTSD, I turned to CrossFit®, a high-intensity functional-training (HIFT) Programme that blends metabolic conditioning, gymnastics, and Olympic lifting (Feito et al., 2018). Preliminary evidence links HIFT to improved mood, fitness, and exercise adherence (Claudino et al., 2018), yet its therapeutic value for PTSD is largely untested, particularly in veteran populations (Ferrer & Davis, 2019).

Theoretical lens: Self-Determination Theory (SDT). SDT posits that psychological well-being flourishes when autonomy, competence, and relatedness are satisfied (Deci & Ryan, 1985; Ryan & Deci, 2017). CrossFit's peer-supported, mastery-oriented culture appears well suited to meet these needs (Kerry, 2017; Teixeira et al., 2012), providing a plausible mechanism through which the Programme might alleviate PTSD symptomatology.

J. Alder, *Military Men, Physical Exercise, and Post-Traumatic Stress Disorder*, Palgrave Studies in Masculinity, Sport and Exercise,
https://doi.org/10.1007/978-3-032-08957-1_4

Autoethnography as method. Autoethnography, melding autobiography with ethnography, places lived experience at the centre of scholarly analysis (Allen-Collinson, 2012; Ritchie, 2019). By documenting my 12-week CrossFit journey through reflective journals and field notes, I offer an insider perspective on how HIFT interacts with PTSD in daily life.

Purpose of the Chapter. Guided by SDT, this autoethnography examines how a CrossFit regimen influenced my autonomy, competence, and relatedness and, in turn, my PTSD symptoms and overall well-being. In addressing the paucity of research on community-based, exercise-oriented interventions for combat veterans (Able & Benedek, 2019; Petz, 2021), the Chapter seeks to generate novel insight and practical guidance for clinicians, coaches, and veterans alike.

Methodology

Philosophical Foundations

The foundations of this Chapter are rooted in interpretivist and constructionist paradigms, which emphasise understanding human behaviour and lived experiences rather than capturing a fixed, objective reality (Avramidis & Smith, 1999; Creswell, 2013). These paradigms suggest that reality is fluid, shaped by context and individual interpretation (Gibson, 2019; Guerrettaz et al., 2021), and that researchers and participants are mutually engaged in the co-construction of knowledge (Creswell, 2014; Fossey et al., 2002).

Aligned with this, the Chapter adopts epistemological constructionism and subjectivism, acknowledging that knowledge is shaped by individual and cultural perceptions (Mills et al., 2006; Palincsar, 1998; Scotland, 2012). In this framework, reality is understood as contingent, subjective, and influenced by social context (Levers, 2013; Van der Walt, 2020). Rather than viewing knowledge as fixed, it is seen as the product of interaction between self, society, and culture (Brown-Jeffy & Cooper, 2011; Poucher et al., 2020; Young & Collin, 2004).

Narrative Inquiry and Autoethnography

Given the multiplicity of perspectives and the absence of a singular truth in social life, this Chapter employs narrative inquiry as its overarching methodological framework (Willig, 2013). Narrative inquiry allows for the exploration of how individuals interpret and give meaning to lived experiences through story (Ellis et al., 2011; Fraser, 2004). Narratives are shaped by both personal beliefs and broader sociocultural forces, acting as a lens through which people organise their realities and engage with the world (Frank, 2013; McAdams & McLean, 2013; Robinson, 2011).

While historically underutilised in sport and exercise psychology, narrative inquiry has shown significant promise in revealing the nuanced experiences of injury, illness, and identity (Smith & Sparkes, 2009; Smith & McGannon, 2018). Through its use of rich, humanistic storytelling, it facilitates broader resonance, applicability, and the construction of meaningful knowledge (Sparkes & Smith, 2014; McChesney & Aldridge, 2019).

Within this paradigm, autoethnography emerges as the central mode of inquiry. As a qualitative method that integrates autobiographical narrative with ethnographic analysis, autoethnography enables researchers to explore cultural experiences through personal reflection (Allen-Collinson, 2012; Anderson, 2006). It challenges traditional notions of objectivity by foregrounding the researcher's own perspective and experiences, thereby repositioning subjectivity as a strength (Smith & Sparkes, 2020; Karnieli-Miller et al., 2009).

Researcher Reflexivity and Insider Role

As both researcher and participant, I adopt a dual role central to the autoethnographic tradition. As a military veteran with lived experience of combat-related PTSD, I offer an insider account of trauma, healing, and meaning-making. This positioning enabled me to access and articulate deeply personal insights that might otherwise remain inaccessible to external observers. At the same time, the act of analysis and theoretical engagement allowed for a critical stance on my own narrative and the broader cultural frameworks surrounding it.

Analytical Position and Narrative Continuum

Autoethnography exists on an evocative–analytical continuum (Jones et al., 2016; McMahon, 2019). Evocative autoethnographies emphasise storytelling and emotional resonance (Bochner & Ellis, 2016), while analytical autoethnographies prioritise theory building and conceptual contribution (Le Roux, 2017). This Chapter adopts a moderate position, blending emotionally engaged narrative with structured theoretical reflection (Stahlke-Wall, 2016; Wall, 2016). This approach aims to connect lived experience with scholarly insight in a manner that is both intellectually rigorous and personally authentic (Smith & Sparkes, 2020).

This methodology is increasingly used in sport and exercise psychology, particularly to investigate issues such as identity, mental health, and embodied experience (Douglas & Carless, 2014; Brown et al., 2009). Despite criticisms that autoethnography may overemphasise the subjective at the expense of broader analysis (Anderson, 2006), its potential to produce deeply meaningful and culturally situated knowledge is increasingly recognised (Mayan, 2023; Tracy, 2019).

Method

Ethical Approval

Ethical clearance was granted and all procedures conformed to the British Psychological Society's Code of Human Research Ethics.

Design and Memory-Based Data Generation

Guided by autoethnography, the Chapter employed memory work—self-reflection, narrative reconstruction, and retrieval of autobiographical memories (Chang, 2016). These techniques, informed by extant literature (Ellis et al., 2011; Smith, 2019), deepened exploration of personal experience and enhanced analytic richness (Chang, 2016; Giorgio, 2016).

Ethical Safeguards

- Informed consent & withdrawal. The Chapter's aims, risks, and voluntary nature were communicated transparently (Giorgio, 2016).
- Confidentiality. Pseudonyms and secure, encrypted storage protected identities (Lapadat, 2017).
- Well-being monitoring. Regular check-ins with supervisory and combat-stress staff mitigated potential distress (Bochner & Ellis, 2016).

Narrative Construction

First-person vignettes were crafted chronologically to evoke sensory detail and emotional tone (Day, 2019; Krane, 2019). Fiction-writing techniques (Carless et al., 2014; Smith, 2019) and vernacular language (Kwon, 2016) helped make events vivid for academic and lay audiences alike.

Trustworthiness and Quality

Autoethnography eschews positivist "verification"; instead, narratives were evaluated against genre-specific criteria—evocation, authenticity, coherence, and resonance (Bochner & Ellis, 2016; Sparkes, 2000). This relativist stance recognises stories as truthful accounts of lived experience (Ellis, 2007).

Researcher Reflexivity

Occupying dual roles of storyteller and analyst (Frank, 2013), I critically examined my assumptions and positionality throughout data generation and interpretation (Allen-Collinson, 2012). Reflexive journal entries, structured with Gibbs's cycle, documented impacts of my military background, PTSD, and power relations on the research process (Malthouse et al., 2014).

Analytic Strategy

- Narrative (content) analysis mapped how I made sense of PTSD and CrossFit®.
- Holistic-form structural analysis inspected plot, sequence, and narrative typology (Tony et al., 2015).
- Findings were interpreted through the lenses of Self-Determination Theory and moderate autoethnographic positioning (Stahlke-Wall, 2016; Wall, 2016).

Quality Checks

Potential data-quality critiques (Livesey & Runsen, 2018; Roy & Uekusa, 2020; Tullis et al., 2009) were addressed via:

- Prolonged engagement with the material;
- Peer debriefing with supervisors;
- Member-like reflections with trusted veterans to ensure experiential resonance.

Transition to Vignettes and Data Analysis

Informed by the methodological stance outlined above, the following section presents three analytic vignettes constructed from my 12-week CrossFit® experience. These narrative fragments draw upon personal memory, field notes, and reflective journaling to explore the psychological processes of trauma recovery through the lens of Self-Determination Theory. Each vignette is followed by a theoretical commentary that critically examines how CrossFit® intersected with PTSD symptom reduction and supported the basic psychological needs of autonomy, competence, and relatedness.

Personal Vignette

8 October 2012—Pirbright Training Camp

CrossFit®? Not for me.

The morning sun spilled through the window at 0700, draping the staff restroom of Pirbright Army Selection Centre in a golden hush. Cradling a mug of coffee, its heat steadying my hands, I tried to still a mind rattled by the night's flashbacks. This room, dim and tiled, was my refuge before the day's orders arrived.

The door swung open and Chris stepped in. Fitness banter was our ritual, a momentary bridge between soldier and civilian. Today he dropped a new word: CrossFit®.

> "Think of it as circuit training", he said, "but with gymnastics and power-lifting mixed in".

I heard only circuit training and shrugged, nothing I hadn't done a hundred times. Chris's tone sharpened; he insisted CrossFit® was different, better. I compared it to Tour de France stage training. He bristled; I laughed. The conversation ended in an awkward silence neither rank nor routine could repair.

Later, over lunch, Chris reignited the debate with evangelic fury. My dismissal, equal parts ignorance and ego sent him stalking out. His absence left a tangible crack in our team's camaraderie, and anxiety pooled in its place.

Chris was a civilian contractor, but within these walls his Programming expertise carried weight. That fact forced me to examine my own boundaries, why was I threatened by a workout routine?

That night, after a gruelling PTSD therapy session, I sought refuge in the empty gym. The clang of plates felt honest in a way conversation hadn't. Still, the unease lingered.

So, I called a muster of sorts: coffee, straight talk, no rank. I apologised to the lads and to Chris for my knee-jerk reaction, then admitted what few knew: I was fighting PTSD. Vulnerability broke the tension faster than rank ever could. Chris flashed a grin and answered with his trademark battle cry— "CrossFit®!"—turning the moment from confession to camaraderie.

Workdays settled back into rhythm. Chris and I still sparred over sports, but a new respect softened the edges. I promised I'd give CrossFit® one honest shot.

Looking back, that restroom standoff now feels like a micro-battle in a larger war, me vs. my own closed defences. Chris's challenge cracked the armour. Through that crack I glimpsed the possibility that new methods and new people could help me reclaim autonomy, rebuild competence, and feel connected again.

Analytic Commentary: Linking Lived Experience to Self-Determination Theory (SDT)

Conflict as a Catalyst for Basic-need Frustration

The restroom confrontation between Chris and me was more than a surface-level squabble about exercise modalities; it represented a moment of basic-need frustration (Ryan & Deci, 2017). My dismissive "Tour de France" quip undermined Chris's sense of competence, while his competitive retort threatened my autonomy as the unit's fitness authority. By foregrounding this tension, the narrative illustrates how everyday frictions in military culture can illuminate SDT's motivational mechanics. In highlighting this link, I invite practitioners to notice similar micro-fractures in their own environments before they widen into disengagement or burnout.

Re-authoring Relatedness

My decision to disclose a PTSD diagnosis during the follow-up group meeting was risky, yet it re-authored the social script from rivalry to solidarity. SDT posits that relatedness is nourished when one feels understood and accepted (Deci & Ryan, 2012). By placing vulnerability at the centre of the narrative, this vignette demonstrates how transparent self-disclosure can convert a potentially volatile environment into a psychologically safe space for growth. Practitioners who supervise or coach veterans may consider replicating this structured "psychological unmasking" to accelerate group cohesion.

Competence Reframed: From Physical Mastery to Emotional Regulation

It would be easy to interpret my subsequent gym session merely as a quest for fitness benchmarks; instead, it served as an auto-regulatory intervention. Each lift and kilometre helped manage sympathetic arousal and re-channel intrusive combat memories. Framing exercise as affect regulation, rather than simply conditioning, elevates competence from a muscular metric to a biopsychosocial asset—aligning with contemporary SDT extensions into well-being science.

Autonomy Within a Hierarchical Setting

Military life is saturated with external regulation. Choosing—even quietly—to "give CrossFit® a try" after the conflict exemplifies autonomy enactment amid hierarchy. This narrative demonstrates how micro-choices (e.g., trialling a new modality, adjusting language when debating peers) can restore self-determination without undermining command structure. This insight is actionable for unit PTIs seeking to integrate veteran agency while maintaining operational discipline.

Implications and Roadmap for Translational Practice

By weaving first-person memory with SDT constructs, this Chapter models a practice-proximal autoethnography that offers a framework for applied sport psychology:

- Recognition: Identify moments when gym banter masks deeper need frustration.
- Disclosure: Use strategic self-sharing to unlock relatedness and destigmatise PTSD.
- Reframing: Coach athletes to view performance metrics as vehicles for emotional mastery.
- Choice architecture: Embed small, self-endorsed decisions within rigid training schedules.

These four steps comprise a portable toolkit for sport psychologists, mental health practitioners, and CrossFit® coaches working with combat veterans.

Reflective Close

Writing and analysing this vignette crystallised a core realisation: my recovery is not solely a private journey but a replicable template. By amplifying the connections between lived conflict, SDT need-satisfaction, and trauma regulation, this autoethnography offers a translational model grounded in both theory and experience. In doing so, it supports the agenda of Psychology of Sport and Exercise to translate robust psychological frameworks into transformative real-world practice.

Personal Vignette

30 January 2020—"Crossing the Rubicon and Starting My CrossFit® Journey"

30 January 2020. A day that would become a turning point in my life. This is the story of my serendipitous encounter with CrossFit®—a journey that would transform my life in unexpected and profound ways.

From the moment I stepped into CrossFit Basin View, I was welcomed into an atmosphere brimming with palpable energy and camaraderie. The space pulsed with an infectious enthusiasm—a place where sweat mingled with determination and the clatter of weights harmonised with the encouraging banter of fellow athletes. The CrossFit® community was bound by a shared commitment to pushing boundaries, radiating a sense of unity and purpose.

I approached with a mixture of excitement and trepidation. The day's workout loomed before me, a complex series of exercises that promised both challenge and exhilaration: box jumps, CrossFit® burpees, assault bike intervals, clean and jerks, power cleans, hang snatches, handstand push-ups, and kipping pull-ups. Each movement felt like a foreign language I was determined to learn.

Amidst this symphony of exertion, I began to absorb a new lexicon—one that would soon become central to my daily life. "Box" referred to this hallowed space of transformation. "WOD", short for Workout of the Day, became my compass. Terms like "For Time", "EMOM" (Every Minute on the Minute), and "AMRAP" (As Many Rounds as Possible) became part of a vocabulary that connected me to this new world.

Surprisingly, I found myself reflecting on Chris, who had once passionately advocated for CrossFit®. He had been right all along. CrossFit® wasn't merely a form of exercise; it was a philosophy. It celebrated resilience, community, and the pursuit of self-betterment. As I moved through the WOD, fuelled by adrenaline and focus, I felt a deep resonance with CrossFit's ethos. Each rep became a testament to breaking past my perceived limits.

Yet fate intervened. Just two months into my training, the COVID-19 pandemic descended. The CrossFit® box, my newfound sanctuary was shuttered. I was left adrift, again. But this time, I responded differently.

Undeterred, I converted my basement into a makeshift gym. It was far from ideal, but it became a haven. Amidst virtual encouragement and distant memories of the box, I kept going. The workouts became my anchor, an antidote to the isolation and uncertainty of the pandemic.

As weeks passed, I experienced a transformation that went far beyond physical gains. CrossFit® evolved into something deeply therapeutic. The clang of weights and the imagined voices of my CrossFit® community became intertwined with a growing sense of hope. Slowly, the grip of anxiety loosened. The intrusive thoughts that once dominated my mornings began to fade.

What shocked me most was the gradual reduction in my reliance on medication and formal therapies. The endorphins, the structure, the sense of agency, all became my new therapy. Each workout reminded me that my body, once a site of trauma, could also be a source of healing.

CrossFit® became more than a workout; it became a way to reclaim control. It redefined my relationship with movement, resilience, and recovery. No longer was I exercising to simply stay fit, I was healing. I was rediscovering myself.

This journey, born in a brightly lit box and continued in a dim basement, marked the beginning of a new chapter. My PTSD symptoms began to recede. In their place: confidence, clarity, and connection. CrossFit® had provided me with the resilience and camaraderie that years of military service had taken from me.

Crossing into the world of CrossFit® transformed my relationship with exercise and became a powerful tool in navigating PTSD. Fuelled by determination and supported by community, even virtually, this journey revealed the resilience of the human spirit. What began as a reluctant step into a CrossFit® box evolved into a healing process that redefined what recovery could mean.

Analytic Commentary: Bringing My Journey into Focus Through Self-Determination Theory

Positioning the Narrative

This second vignette is more than a fitness memoir; it is an autoethnographic test case showing how the three basic needs in Self-Determination Theory (SDT)—autonomy, competence, and relatedness—can be met in ways that loosen the grip of combat-related PTSD (Ryan & Deci, 2017). By mapping each turning point in my CrossFit® experience onto these mechanisms, I provide an evidence-in-action blueprint that veterans, coaches, and clinicians can adapt. I write as both scholar and survivor to underscore how personal agency and theory can co-produce recovery.

Autonomy: Reclaiming Choice Under Lockdown Constraints

Crossing the Basin View threshold on 30 January 2020 was the first decisive act of self-endorsement I had made since leaving active duty. No one ordered me to train; I initiated the change, chose the box, and embraced the unfamiliar language of WODs and EMOMs. SDT predicts that such self-directed choices restore a sense of volition often stripped away by regimented military life and the vigilance demanded by PTSD (Deci & Ryan, 2012). My later decision to keep training alone in a basement gym, rather than surrendering to pandemic inertia, shows how micro-acts of choice can safeguard autonomy even when external freedoms shrink.

Take-home for practice: Help trauma-affected athletes author at least one training variable (location, timing, load, or movement selection); even a small decision can reignite control.

Competence: Redefining Mastery as Emotional Regulation

Each assault-bike interval became less about wattage and more about controlling arousal. I learned to transform the surge of a clean and jerk into a deliberate exposure exercise, mirroring cognitive-behavioural principles. Thus, my sense of competence shifted from chasing external performance metrics to cultivating internal regulation skills (Ryan & Deci, 2008). As load and skill improved, so did my ability to down-regulate intrusive memories and panic cues—paralleling findings that physical mastery can enhance emotion regulation in PTSD populations (Ferrer & Davis, 2019).

Take-home for practice: Recast PRs (personal records) as **PRRs—personal regulation records—**where the benchmark is post-session affect, sleep quality, or reduced reliance on medication.

Relatedness: Community Beyond the Box

When COVID-19 closed the gym, virtual high-fives and WhatsApp check-ins preserved the feeling of being seen and valued. Those digital echoes sustained the belonging that SDT identifies as essential for motivation and well-being (Johnston & Finney, 2010). In a disorder marked by withdrawal, that thread of connection was literally life-saving. Research on veteran integration confirms that peer support can buffer against isolation and relapse (Caddick & Smith, 2014; Lundberg et al., 2011).

Take-home for practice: Coaches can foster "ambient relatedness" (leader boards, voice-note encouragement) when in-person contact is impossible; the signal of belonging matters more than the medium.

Translational Significance for PTSD Recovery

By weaving first-person narrative with SDT constructs, I model a practice-proximal pathway that others can replicate:

- Autonomy prompts—invite veterans to author meaningful elements of each session.
- Competence reframing—track self-regulation gains, not just weight lifted.
- Relatedness scaffolds—create micro-rituals of support that survive lockdowns or deployments.

Together, these steps form a portable toolkit for deploying CrossFit® (or any functional fitness modality) as an adjunct to PTSD treatment.

Concluding Reflection: From Single Story to Shared Protocol

My basement burpees were not a solitary triumph; they are proof that SDT-informed training can convert exercise into exposure, mastery, and reconnection—three pillars of trauma recovery. By narrating and analysing these moments side by side, I invite fellow veterans to recognise their own turning points and equip practitioners with a theoretically grounded, experientially validated roadmap. In advancing this dialogue, the commentary aligns with the Psychology of Sport and Exercise mission to translate robust theory into transformative practice.

Personal Vignette

2 October 2021—"A Journey of Redemption: Healing Through the CrossFit® Community"

During the turbulent upheavals brought about by the COVID-19 lockdowns, the highly anticipated reopening of the CrossFit® box in early October 2021 could not have come soon enough. That day marked more than a return to structured physical training—it was a symbolic reclaiming of the shattered fragments of my mental well-being. The closures had not only confined me physically but reopened deep scars of PTSD, etched into my psyche from my time in Iraq.

The isolation that came with lockdown acted as a cruel echo chamber, amplifying my trauma and triggering waves of tormenting symptoms—vivid flashbacks, surging anxiety, simmering anger, the heavy grip of depression, and a desolate emotional numbness. Solitude became fertile ground for intrusive memories, which resurfaced with a raw, unrelenting intensity. At times, I was barely able to hold on to a thread of stability.

And yet, amidst the silence, a glimmer of hope emerged. The day the CrossFit® box flung open its doors marked the intersection of physical return and emotional reawakening—a personal odyssey towards healing, growth, and redemption.

The familiar clang of weights, the soft thud of skipping ropes, and the sharp scent of rubber mats instantly grounded me. The sensory overload was powerful but strangely reassuring—here was a place where I could fight back, repurpose my pain, and reclaim control. The sheer intensity of the workouts offered a much-needed release valve, allowing me to channel the frustration and anguish that had festered during months of enforced isolation.

But it wasn't just the movements that brought relief.

As I immersed myself in those sweat-drenched sessions, a deeper transformation began to unfold. The camaraderie with my fellow athletes shifted from friendly banter to something more profound—a lifeline. It became a tether that held me steady as I fought my internal battles. The shared exhaustion, the unified struggle, the simple nods of encouragement—they wrapped around me like armour. Together, they formed a protective barrier against the chaos raging inside.

This reconnection offered me something I hadn't felt in years: identity and purpose. What had been stripped away by war and isolation was now being rebuilt through collective effort and belonging. Brick by brick, my resilience was being restored.

This healing wasn't immediate. It was hard-earned—lift by lift, breath by breath, set by set. But it was real.

The most profound moment came when I noticed I was relying less on the medications and therapies that had once seemed essential. The endorphin-fuelled highs of CrossFit®, the consistency of effort, and the meaning found in each session began to replace what traditional treatments could not fully reach. The box became more than a gym. It became a sanctuary.

My journey, intertwined with the CrossFit® community, stands as a powerful testament to transformation. From the depths of despair shaped by PTSD, I emerged not only with renewed strength and hope but with an unbreakable connection to a group of people who unknowingly saved me. Through the laughter, the sweat, the shared adversity, I found something vital: the path to healing runs through connection. And that path is made not just in silence or solitude, but in the shouted encouragement of a partner beside you, in the sound of a rig slapping back into place, in the gritty breath of the final rep.

The CrossFit® box, once merely a place for physical exertion, became a crucible where I reforged my fractured self. In the presence of those who understood struggle—not always through words but through effort—I found a way to reframe my pain and reclaim my story.

Analytic Commentary: Reflective Analysis of Healing Through CrossFit® and Self-Determination Theory

This section presents a critically reflective account of my re-entry into the CrossFit® community through the lens of Self-Determination Theory (SDT)—a well-established psychological framework that posits autonomy, competence, and relatedness as essential for human motivation, growth, and well-being (Ryan & Deci, 2000, 2017). While grounded in personal experience, this narrative serves as an autoethnographic exemplar that illustrates how CrossFit® functioned not only as a space for physical rehabilitation but also as a trauma-responsive intervention during my ongoing recovery from combat-related PTSD.

Healing and Redemption Through the CrossFit® Community

On 2 October 2021, I stepped back into the CrossFit® box for the first time since the COVID-19 lockdowns began. This was more than the reopening of a gym—it marked a symbolic and psychological threshold: a return to community, to structure, and most importantly, to self-directed healing. Through the lens of SDT, this moment represented a reassertion of autonomy: a choice to re-engage on my own terms after months of stagnation and psychological contraction (Deci & Ryan, 2012; Patrick & Williams, 2012).

Autonomy, in this context, wasn't simply about picking exercises. It was about choosing how to confront fear, how to set limits, and how to re-establish identity after the twin traumas of PTSD and pandemic isolation. Veterans often experience a loss of agency due to rigid military systems and the psychological grip of trauma (Noori, 2020; Hornby, 2015). My decision to return to CrossFit®—to navigate workouts, scale my challenges, and reintegrate socially—became a powerful expression of reclaimed personal control.

Transformation and Resilience Through Competence and Relatedness

Inside the gym, I pushed through assault-bike intervals and Olympic lifts, but what I gained was far beyond fitness. CrossFit® became a vehicle for emotional regulation. Each session helped me harness adrenaline, reduce intrusive thoughts, and build psychophysiological control—a key therapeutic goal in PTSD treatment (Van Gelderen et al., 2018; Dominski et al., 2021). My sense of competence no longer hinged on hitting PRs (personal records) but on post-session calm, better sleep, and reduced medication reliance.

Equally transformative was the experience of relatedness. Post-WOD fist bumps, shared grunts of exhaustion, and side comments during rest intervals were small gestures that rebuilt trust and connection, both essential antidotes to the isolating effects of trauma (Johnston & Finney, 2010). These bonds required no disclosure of my PTSD. Instead, the relational rhythm of the box—the slap of barbells on rubber, the sour-sweet smell of sweat and steel, and the affirming cheers during AMRAPs—created a safe relational space. This unspoken solidarity restored a sense of social belonging, eroded by years of hypervigilance and emotional withdrawal (Caddick & Smith, 2014).

CrossFit® as Trauma-Informed Practice: Translating SDT into Action

By aligning lived experience with SDT principles, the following table outlines how my CrossFit® journey maps onto evidence-based recovery strategies for PTSD:

Table 4.1 outlines the principles of trauma-informed physical activity. This integrative approach is supported by recent scholarship advocating for trauma-informed physical activity that centres autonomy, co-regulation, and safety (Treleaven, 2018).

Table 4.1 Turning theory into practice: SDT in action

SDT need	*What I did*	*Trauma-informed strategy*
Autonomy	Chose my WOD structure, pace, and environment	Encouraged agency and reduced helplessness
Competence	Reframed goals around emotional regulation	Built mastery and reduced fear-based avoidance behaviours
Relatedness	Reconnected through shared routines and support	Countered social withdrawal and enhanced safety through bonds

Note. WOD = Workout of the Day; SDT = Self-Determination Theory

Conclusion: Rebuilding a Life, Not Just a Body

This reflective narrative highlights how structured physical activity, when guided by SDT and embedded in a supportive community, can catalyse meaningful psychological change. CrossFit® became more than a fitness regimen; it was a reparative framework—a site where I could redefine myself not by symptoms or service history, but by agency, resilience, and human connection (Ryan & Deci, 2017; Heintzelman, 2018).

While this is my story, it offers a replicable blueprint for coaches, clinicians, and veterans seeking trauma-informed, theory-grounded pathways to recovery. It calls for sport and exercise professionals to recognise that healing happens in relationship—to movement, to others, and most importantly, to the self.

Personal Vignette

3 March 2023—"A Race to Normal Life: Healing Through CrossFit® Programming"

3 March 2023. A date etched into my memory, the moment my life began to shift from merely surviving with PTSD to reclaiming a sense of self. What began as a physical endeavour soon evolved into a transformative experience. This is the story of how a structured CrossFit® Programme became a turning point in my journey towards recovery.

At that time, I was burdened by the weight of trauma, hypervigilance, nightmares, emotional withdrawal. The world felt fragmented, and my grip on stability had become increasingly fragile. Yet within this chaos emerged a sense of clarity: I needed structure, community, and purpose—elements I had once found in uniform and now hoped to rediscover through movement.

The scent of rubber mats and chalk hit me as I stepped into the gym. The clang of bumper plates and the slap of the rig sparked a visceral memory—not of war zones, but of hard-won focus. I had joined CrossFit® before, but this time was different. I was no longer just attending workouts. I was about to commit to a 12-week personalised Programme designed in collaboration with Alan, a Level 3 CrossFit® coach. It wasn't just about fitness—it was a calculated intervention, a bid to reclaim my agency and reduce my reliance on medication.

Each session became a deliberate act of resistance against PTSD's grip. I tracked the highs and lows—how I felt post-WOD, how I slept, whether nightmares came. Week by week, the changes weren't just physical. The anxiety that had felt like a shadow at my shoulder began to retreat. The flashbacks that once held me hostage lost their edge. Even my temper, once volatile and ever-present, softened into something I could manage. CrossFit® wasn't curing me, but it was helping me rebuild.

One of the most powerful shifts was internal. With every lift, sprint, and stretch, I found myself growing and not just in strength, but in confidence. I no longer measured success in pounds or seconds, but in calmness, connection, and control. What had once seemed like impossible obstacles, crowded spaces, unexpected noises, vulnerability, were now manageable. They had become part of the workout, not threats to be avoided.

Equally vital was the environment around me. The CrossFit® community, without knowing the details of my trauma, became a support system. Shared effort, mutual encouragement, and silent understanding created a psychological safety net. I didn't have to explain, I simply had to show up, be present, and sweat beside others. And that, somehow, was enough.

Perhaps the most significant realisation came quietly. One day, I faced a known PTSD trigger. My heart rate spiked, but I stayed present. I used the same breathing I practised on the rower. And I noticed: the fear had lessened. I was no longer being pulled under by my past—I was rising above it. That moment marked a turning point. CrossFit® had become a toolkit, equipping me not just to perform, but to heal.

Looking back, the 12-week Programme wasn't just about programming. It was about transformation. I emerged from that period not "cured", but reconnected—with my body, my mind, and my life. The weights didn't just build muscle—they rebuilt my confidence. The workouts didn't just push my limits—they reshaped my narrative.

CrossFit® became the container that held my suffering, channelled my rage, and offered me a way back to myself. For those of us living with trauma, this type of training can offer more than strength, it provides structure, purpose, and, ultimately, hope.

Analytic Commentary: CrossFit® as a Catalyst for Autonomy, Healing, and PTSD Recovery

This analytic reflection demonstrates how CrossFit® did not simply support my PTSD recovery—it actively transformed it. More than offering momentary relief, it became a consistent, structured practice through which I regained control over my symptoms. Framed through Self-Determination Theory (SDT), this journey evidences how the psychological needs of autonomy, competence, and relatedness were not only reawakened but mobilised to deliver meaningful and lasting relief from combat-related trauma.

Autonomy Regained: Turning Choice into Power

PTSD had confined my life to patterns of avoidance, medication, and emotional shutdown. On 3 March 2023, I deliberately chose to begin a 12-week CrossFit® Programme. This was more than a fitness decision—it was an act of defiance against the inertia of trauma. That decision—to self-direct my healing—reinstated personal agency, a key SDT mechanism (Deci & Ryan, 2012).

Crucially, CrossFit® gave me back control: I could tailor the movements, scale the load, and define progress in ways that felt right for me. This autonomy allowed me to actively confront my condition, not passively manage it. I was no longer merely coping with PTSD; I was reshaping my daily experience in ways that reduced symptoms and increased psychological freedom (Ryan et al., 2019).

Competence: Training the Body, Mastering the Mind

As the weeks progressed, I discovered that the weight I was lifting was only half the story. What mattered more was how I used those sessions to master my inner state. CrossFit® became my exposure therapy, allowing me to confront triggers, regulate arousal, and build emotional stability—one rep, one breath, one WOD at a time.

By week six, I was no longer tracking physical gains alone. I was measuring competence through deeper sleep, fewer intrusive thoughts, and the radical shift in no longer needing medication to manage daily symptoms. My training became a tool for psychological self-regulation—evidence that I was in charge of my recovery, not at the mercy of it (Ryan & Deci, 2008; Dominski et al., 2021).

Relatedness: Connection That Heals

Lockdown isolation and the aftermath of military service had carved a gulf between me and others. The CrossFit® box filled that void. The micro-interactions—encouragement from my coach, shared effort with others, silent nods of respect—began to rebuild a sense of social trust. I didn't need to explain my trauma for this community to support me. Their presence was enough (Caddick & Smith, 2014).

In SDT terms, this fulfilled my need for relatedness, giving me the psychological safety and connection necessary for sustained motivation and emotional healing. CrossFit® became more than a gym—it became a lifeline.

Structured Freedom: A Blueprint for Recovery

By the end of the 12-week Programme, the gains were no longer just physical. I had experienced a significant reduction in PTSD symptoms, a complete break from medication, and a renewed capacity to engage with life. Autonomy, competence, and relatedness had formed a synergistic recovery loop—CrossFit® didn't just supplement therapy; in many ways, it outperformed it.

This is not anecdotal; it is lived evidence. For veterans, coaches, and clinicians, the implications are clear: CrossFit®—when intentionally structured—can serve as an adjunctive, even primary, recovery modality. Below is a practice-informed model of how SDT mechanisms were activated during this process:

Table 4.2 illustrates how Self-Determination Theory (SDT) mechanisms are activated in CrossFit® and their impact on PTSD recovery. This evidence highlights how autonomy, competence, and relatedness can

Table 4.2 Activation of Self-Determination Theory mechanisms in CrossFit® and their impact on PTSD recovery

SDT need	*Applied mechanism in CrossFit®*	*PTSD recovery outcome*
Autonomy	Choosing pace, movement type, session timing	Increased control, reduced helplessness
Competence	Reframing progress as emotional regulation	Less anxiety, better sleep, no medication
Relatedness	Supportive environment, consistent encouragement	Rebuilt trust, increased motivation

Note. SDT = Self-Determination Theory; PTSD = Post-Traumatic Stress Disorder.

foster increased control, reduced helplessness, emotional regulation, improved sleep, and enhanced motivation.

Chapter Conclusion

This chapter has traced a deeply personal yet widely relevant trajectory of trauma recovery, where physical exercise, specifically CrossFit®, functioned not simply as a fitness regime but as a therapeutic intervention grounded in the principles of Self-Determination Theory (SDT). Through the lens of lived experience, it has demonstrated that CrossFit® offered more than symptom relief; it provided the structure, agency, and community necessary to reclaim a life interrupted by post-traumatic stress disorder.

At the heart of this recovery was the restoration of autonomy. Re-entering the CrossFit® box as a veteran with PTSD was not an act of casual participation, but a conscious reclaiming of personal power. Each decision, whether to scale a workout, confront a fear, or simply show up, reasserted control in a context where control had long been lost. This experience validates SDT's premise that autonomy is foundational to motivation and mental health (Deci & Ryan, 1985; Ryan & Deci, 2000). In regaining the right to choose how to engage with my body and emotions, I became the author of my own recovery.

Competence followed, not just through progressive physical achievements but through enhanced emotional resilience. Activities that initially triggered hyperarousal or avoidance gradually transformed into opportunities for regulation, growth, and reflection. Monitoring my reactions across the 12-week Programme evidenced a decline in classic PTSD symptoms such as flashbacks, intrusive thoughts, and heightened vigilance.

These were replaced by an emerging sense of capability. I was no longer at the mercy of my trauma; I was actively learning to navigate it.

The third dimension, relatedness, was perhaps the most unexpected but profound. In a military context where masculine ideals often constrain emotional expression and recovery, the CrossFit® community offered an alternative model of masculinity. This was one rooted in mutual respect, shared struggle, and vulnerability through effort. Connection came not through confession but through consistency. The presence of others who stood beside me, unconditionally, helped to dismantle the isolation that had taken hold during both deployment and civilian life. This sense of belonging proved as healing as any formal therapy.

CrossFit® did not provide a cure. What it did provide, crucially, were the tools and environment in which I could re-engage with life. I was not a passive recipient of clinical treatment but an empowered participant in my own recovery. It allowed me to reconnect with a version of masculinity that embraced strength without stoicism, effort without ego, and vulnerability without shame.

The broader implications of this chapter invite a reimagining of PTSD interventions for veterans and others affected by trauma. Clinical approaches often overlook the psychosocial dimensions of healing. By contrast, this narrative highlights how a community-based exercise model grounded in SDT can address precisely those domains: autonomy, competence, and relatedness. These are essential to holistic recovery. The reduction in reliance on pharmacological solutions, the improvements in sleep and emotional regulation, and the renewed sense of identity all point to the transformative potential of integrating physical activity into mental health care.

This chapter is not without limitations. It is, unapologetically, a subjective account. Yet in this subjectivity lies its strength. By offering an embodied narrative, it invites further research, reflection, and replication. It challenges dominant models of hypermasculine suppression within both military and therapeutic cultures. It also suggests that healing can be found not in silence, but in sweat; not in retreat, but in reconnection.

In closing, CrossFit® did not rescue me in a romanticised or metaphorical sense. It gave me back what trauma had taken: the capacity to act, to feel, to relate, and to grow. It offered relief from the chaos of PTSD. It gave me control over my body and mind. And most powerfully, it offered me the chance to reclaim my life, rep by rep, breath by breath, day by day.

References

Able, M. L., & Benedek, D. M. (2019). Posttraumatic stress disorder in military veterans: A review of prevalence and treatment. *Journal of Military Medicine, 184*(5–6), e223–e230.

Allen-Collinson, J. (2012). Autoethnography: Situating personal sporting narratives in socio-cultural contexts. In K. Young & M. Atkinson (Eds.), *Qualitative research on sport and physical culture* (pp. 191–212). Emerald.

Anderson, L. (2006). Analytic autoethnography. *Journal of Contemporary Ethnography, 35*(4), 373–395.

Avramidis, E., & Smith, B. (1999). An introduction to the major research paradigms and their methodological approaches. *Educational Research Review, 1*(1), 1–20.

Bochner, A. P., & Ellis, C. (2016). *Evocative autoethnography: Writing lives and telling stories.* Routledge.

Brown, T., Jones, R. L., & Holloway, I. (2009). Qualitative research in sport and physical activity: Critical reflections. *European Physical Education Review, 15*(3), 255–272.

Brown-Jeffy, S., & Cooper, J. E. (2011). Toward a conceptual framework of culturally relevant pedagogy. *Teacher Education Quarterly, 38*(1), 65–84.

Caddick, N., & Smith, B. (2014). The impact of sport and physical activity on the well-being of combat veterans: A systematic review. *Psychology of Sport and Exercise, 15*(1), 9–18.

Carless, D., Sparkes, A. C., Douglas, K., & Cooke, C. (2014). Disability, inclusive sport and self-identity: A qualitative study. *Psychology of Sport and Exercise, 15*(1), 196–204.

Chang, H. (2016). *Autoethnography as method.* Routledge.

Claudino, J. G., Gabbett, T. J., Bourgeois, F., Souza, H. S., Miranda, R. C., Mezêncio, B., Soncin, R., Cardoso Filho, C. A., Bottaro, M., Hernandez, A. J., Amadio, A. C., & Serrão, J. C. (2018). CrossFit®: Risk and benefits to participants. *Sports Medicine, 48*(3), 233–252.

Creswell, J. W. (2013). *Qualitative inquiry and research design: Choosing among five approaches* (3rd ed.). Sage.

Creswell, J. W. (2014). *Research design: Qualitative, quantitative, and mixed methods approaches* (4th ed.). Sage.

Day, M. C. (2019). Qualitative inquiry in sport and exercise psychology. *Qualitative Research in Sport, Exercise and Health, 11*(4), 515–518.

Deci, E. L., & Ryan, R. M. (1985). *Intrinsic motivation and self-determination in human behaviour.* Springer.

Deci, E. L., & Ryan, R. M. (2012). Motivation, personality, and development within embedded social contexts: An overview of self-determination theory. In

R. M. Ryan (Ed.), *The Oxford handbook of human motivation* (pp. 85–107). Oxford University Press.

Dominski, F. H., Siqueira, T. C., & Serafim, T. T. (2021). Physical activity and PTSD: Mechanisms and therapeutic potential. *Frontiers in Psychology, 12*, 700–715.

Douglas, K., & Carless, D. (2014). Life story research in sport: Understanding the experiences of elite and professional athletes. *Qualitative Research in Sport, Exercise and Health, 6*(2), 268–277.

Ellis, C. (2007). Telling secrets, revealing lives: Relational ethics in research with intimate others. *Qualitative Inquiry, 13*(1), 3–29.

Ellis, C., Adams, T. E., & Bochner, A. P. (2011). Autoethnography: An overview. Forum: Qualitative. *Social Research, 12*(1), 1–17.

Feito, Y., Heinrich, K. M., Butcher, S. J., & Poston, W. S. (2018). High-intensity functional training (HIFT): Definition and research implications for improved fitness. *Sports, 6*(3), 76–88.

Ferrer, D. A., & Davis, R. W. (2019). Evidence-based physical activity for PTSD and depression in veterans. *Military Medicine, 184*(1–2), e81–e89.

Fossey, E., Harvey, C., McDermott, F., & Davidson, L. (2002). Understanding and evaluating qualitative research. *Australian and New Zealand Journal of Psychiatry, 36*(6), 717–732.

Frank, A. W. (2013). *The wounded storyteller: Body, illness, and ethics* (2nd ed.). University of Chicago Press.

Fraser, M. T. (2004). Autoethnography as research method. *Qualitative Social Work, 3*(4), 359–376.

Gibson, W. J. (2019). Understanding interpretivism. *Qualitative Methods in Psychology Bulletin, 28*(2), 15–20.

Giorgio, G. (2016). Reflections on writing through memory in autoethnography. *Qualitative Inquiry, 22*(9), 699–704.

Guerrettaz, A. M., Zahner, W., & Tenenbaum, G. (2021). Constructionism and its applications in sport psychology. *Sport, Exercise, and Performance Psychology, 10*(3), 320–333.

Heintzelman, S. J. (2018). Eudaimonia in the contemporary science of well-being: Perspectives on psychological well-being and meaning in life. *Research in Human Development, 15*(2), 147–156.

Hornby, G. (2015). Inclusive education: Development, perspectives and challenges. *British Journal of Special Education, 42*(3), 221–239.

Johnston, M., & Finney, S. (2010). Social support and health in military veterans. *Journal of Health Psychology, 15*(2), 117–128.

Jones, S. H., Adams, T. E., & Ellis, C. (2016). *Handbook of autoethnography*. Routledge.

Karnieli-Miller, O., Strier, R., & Pessach, L. (2009). Power relations in qualitative research. *Qualitative Health Research, 19*(2), 279–289.

Kerry, D. S. (2017). Communities of practice and CrossFit®: Cultivating relatedness in sport. *Journal of Sport and Social Issues, 41*(3), 207–225.

Krane, V. (2019). Gendered lives in sport: Qualitative inquiry. *Sport and Exercise Psychology Review, 15*(2), 46–52.

Kwon, J. (2016). Writing with the body: Autoethnography, memory, and trauma. *Qualitative Inquiry, 22*(4), 270–277.

Lapadat, J. C. (2017). Ethics in autoethnography and collaborative autoethnography. *Qualitative Inquiry, 23*(8), 589–603.

Le Roux, C. S. (2017). Analytic autoethnography: Paradigmatic and methodological developments. *International Journal of Qualitative Methods, 16*(1), 1–9.

Levers, M. D. (2013). Philosophical paradigms, grounded theory, and perspectives on emergence. *Sage Open, 3*(4), 1–6.

Livesey, L., & Runsen, H. (2018). Establishing quality in qualitative research: Strategies for trustworthiness. *Qualitative Research in Sport, Exercise and Health, 10*(2), 135–150.

Lundberg, N. R., Bennett, J. L., & Smith, S. (2011). Outcomes of adaptive sports for veterans with PTSD. *Therapeutic Recreation Journal, 45*(2), 105–120.

Malthouse, R., Roffey-Barentsen, J., & Watts, M. (2014). Reflectivity, reflexivity, and situated reflective practice. *Teacher Education Advancement Network Journal, 6*(1), 21–31.

Mayan, M. J. (2023). *Qualitative research: The essential guide to theory and practice* (2nd ed.). Routledge.

McAdams, D. P., & McLean, K. C. (2013). Narrative identity. *Current Directions in Psychological Science, 22*(3), 233–238.

McChesney, K., & Aldridge, J. M. (2019). Narratives of resilience in sport and education. *Sport, Education and Society, 24*(1), 1–12.

McMahon, J. (2019). Autoethnography in sport research. *Qualitative Research in Sport, Exercise and Health, 11*(2), 212–229.

Mills, G., Bonner, A., & Francis, K. (2006). The development of constructivist grounded theory. *International Journal of Qualitative Methods, 5*(1), 25–35.

Noori, A. (2020). Autonomy in military veterans with PTSD. *Journal of Military Psychology, 32*(3), 201–213.

Palincsar, A. S. (1998). Social constructivist perspectives on teaching and learning. *Annual Review of Psychology, 49*(1), 345–375.

Patrick, H., & Williams, G. C. (2012). Self-determination theory: Implications for health behaviour and well-being. *Health Education, 112*(2), 176–180.

Petz, M. R. (2021). Examining the contributions of grit, mental toughness, and conscientiousness to athletic performance [Doctoral dissertation, Capella University].

Poucher, Z. A., Tamminen, K. A., Caron, J. G., & Sweet, S. N. (2020). Thinking through and designing qualitative research studies: A focus on reflexivity. *International Journal of Sport and Exercise Psychology, 18*(2), 111–126.

Ritchie, M. (2019). An autoethnography on the geography of PTSD. *Journal of Loss and Trauma, 24*(1), 69–83.
Robinson, L. (2011). Soldiers' stories of the Falklands War: Recomposing trauma in memoir. *Contemporary British History, 25*(4), 569–589.
Roy, R., & Uekusa, S. (2020). Collaborative autoethnography: "Self-reflection" as a timely alternative research approach during the global pandemic. *Qualitative Research Journal, 20*(4), 383–392.
Ryan, R. M., & Deci, E. L. (2000). Self-determination theory and the facilitation of intrinsic motivation, social development, and well-being. *American Psychologist, 55*(1), 68–78.
Ryan, R. M., & Deci, E. L. (2008). From ego depletion to vitality: Theory and findings concerning the facilitation of energy available to the self. *Social and Personality Psychology Compass, 2*(2), 702–717.
Ryan, R. M., & Deci, E. L. (2017). *Self-determination theory: Basic psychological needs in motivation, development, and wellness.* Guilford Press.
Ryan, R. M., Soenens, B., & Vansteenkiste, M. (2019). Reflections on self-determination theory as an organising framework for personality psychology. *Journal of Personality, 87*(1), 115–145.
Scotland, J. (2012). Exploring the philosophical underpinnings of research: Relating ontology and epistemology to the methodology and methods of the scientific, interpretive, and critical research paradigms. *English Language Teaching, 5*(9), 9–16.
Smith, B. (2019). Narrative analysis in sport and exercise: How can it be done? In B. Smith & A. C. Sparkes (Eds.), *Routledge handbook of qualitative research in sport and exercise* (pp. 260–273). Routledge.
Smith, B., & McGannon, K. R. (2018). Developing rigour in qualitative research: Problems and opportunities within sport and exercise psychology. *International Review of Sport and Exercise Psychology, 11*(1), 101–121.
Smith, B., & Sparkes, A. C. (2009). Narrative inquiry in sport and exercise psychology: What can it mean, and why might we do it? *Psychology of Sport and Exercise, 10*(1), 1–11.
Smith, B., & Sparkes, A. C. (2020). *Qualitative research methods in sport, exercise and health: From process to product.* Routledge.
Sparkes, A. C. (2000). Autoethnography and narratives of self: Reflections on criteria in action. *Sociology of Sport Journal, 17*(1), 21–43.
Sparkes, A. C., & Smith, B. (2014). *Qualitative research methods in sport, exercise and health: From process to product.* Routledge.
Stahlke-Wall, S. (2016). Toward a moderate autoethnography. *International Journal of Qualitative Methods, 15*(1), 1609406916674966.
Teixeira, P. J., Carraça, E. V., Markland, D., Silva, M. N., & Ryan, R. M. (2012). Exercise, physical activity, and self-determination theory: A systematic review.

International Journal of Behavioural Nutrition and Physical Activity, 9(1), 1–30.

Tony, A. E., Jones, S. H., & Ellis, C. (2015). Autoethnography. In J. A. Smith (Ed.), *Understanding qualitative research* (pp. 173–190). Oxford University Press.

Tracy, S. J. (2019). *Qualitative research methods: Collecting evidence, crafting analysis, communicating impact.* Wiley-Blackwell.

Treleaven, D. A. (2018). *Trauma-sensitive mindfulness: Practices for safe and transformative healing.* Norton.

Tullis, J. A., Owen, J. A., McRae, C., Adams, T. E., & Vitale, A. (2009). Truth troubles. *Qualitative Inquiry, 15*(1), 178–200.

Van der Walt, J. L. (2020). Interpretivism–constructivism as a research method in the humanities and social sciences. *International Journal of Philosophy and Theology, 8*(1), 59–68.

Van Gelderen, M. J., Nijdam, M. J., & Vermetten, E. (2018). An innovative framework for delivering psychotherapy to patients with treatment-resistant PTSD: Rationale for interactive motion-assisted therapy. *Frontiers in Psychiatry, 9*, 176–185.

Wall, S. S. (2016). Toward a moderate autoethnography. *International Journal of Qualitative Methods, 15*(1), 1–9.

Willig, C. (2013). *Introducing qualitative research in psychology* (3rd ed.). McGraw-Hill Education.

Young, R. A., & Collin, A. (2004). Introduction: Constructivism and social constructionism in the career field. *Journal of Vocational Behaviour, 64*(3), 373–388.

CHAPTER 5

Exploring the Role of Physical Exercise in the Treatment of PTSD Among Military Veterans

Physical activity is widely acknowledged as a fundamental aspect of cardiovascular fitness and overall well-being (McArdle et al., 2010; Patel et al., 2017). It encompasses various exercise modalities, such as aerobic exercise, anaerobic activity, flexibility training, and functional exercise, each offering distinct benefits to physical and mental health (Hegberg et al., 2019; Herbert et al., 2020).

Before exploring the effects of these exercise modalities on individuals with Post-Traumatic Stress Disorder (PTSD), it is important to provide a brief definition or explanation of PTSD (Andreasen, 2010; Armour et al., 2016). PTSD is a psychological condition that occurs in individuals who have experienced or witnessed a traumatic event, leading to a range of symptoms, including intrusive memories, hypervigilance, and avoidance behaviours (Livingston et al., 2021). Understanding the significance of physical activity and the challenges faced by individuals with PTSD, this Chapter aims to investigate the effectiveness and feasibility of selected exercise modalities as potential treatments for PTSD (Adler & Sipos, 2018; Armour et al., 2015).

J. Alder, *Military Men, Physical Exercise, and Post-Traumatic Stress Disorder*, Palgrave Studies in Masculinity, Sport and Exercise,
https://doi.org/10.1007/978-3-032-08957-1_5

Aerobic Exercise

Several studies have investigated the potential impact of physical activity on individuals with PTSD, with a particular focus on aerobic exercises like walking, running, and swimming (Stults-Kolehmainen & Sinha, 2014; Hegberg et al., 2019). Aerobic exercise, as defined by McArdle et al. (2010), involves the continuous and rhythmic contraction of large muscle groups to Utilise oxygen for energy, aligning with the term "aerobic", which signifies "with oxygen" and relates to the metabolic process of burning fats and carbohydrates in the presence of oxygen.

Incorporating aerobic exercise into a comprehensive fitness Programme, alongside activities such as walking and running, has been considered essential for managing PTSD symptoms (O'Donovan et al., 2010). Additionally, O'Donovan et al. (2010) emphasised the role of a holistic fitness regime encompassing weight training, flexibility exercises, balance drills, and aerobic exercises like walking, running, and swimming in promoting overall health and well-being.

However, it's crucial to acknowledge the limitations of the evidence supporting the efficacy of aerobic exercise for managing PTSD. Some studies have reported mixed results, with variations in the degree of symptom improvement or even symptom exacerbation (Smith et al., 2020). Furthermore, uncertainties persist regarding the optimal duration and intensity of aerobic exercise interventions, owing to variations in Chapter protocols and participant characteristics (Van der Kolk et al., 2020).

To gain a better understanding of the specific mechanisms and optimal parameters for effectively reducing PTSD symptoms through aerobic exercise, further research is warranted (McArdle et al., 2010; Patel et al., 2017). Researchers need to explore factors contributing to mixed results and consider the heterogeneity among individuals with PTSD, Chapter design nuances, and the potential interplay between exercise intensity, duration, and individual response.

Some studies have reported mixed results, with some individuals showing minimal improvement or even experiencing symptom exacerbation (Kurowski et al., 2017; Smith et al., 2020). Moreover, uncertainties persist regarding the optimal duration and intensity of aerobic exercise interventions for individuals with PTSD, as studies have employed varying protocols (Stonerock et al., 2015; Van der Kolk et al., 2020). Therefore, further research is needed to gain a better understanding of the specific mechanisms and optimal parameters for effectively reducing PTSD symptoms through aerobic exercise (Oppizzi & Umberger, 2018; Patel et al., 2017).

Anaerobic Exercise

Anaerobic exercises, such as weightlifting, resistance training, and sprinting, have gained attention as potential therapeutic interventions for individuals with PTSD (Whitworth et al., 2019). These exercises aim to enhance muscle strength and power, providing benefits that extend beyond functional health and beyond cardiovascular fitness (Smith & Merwin, 2021). However, the evidence base regarding the effects of anaerobic exercise on PTSD symptoms requires critical examination (Arent et al., 2020). Currently, the literature on this topic is limited, with few studies specifically examining the impact of anaerobic exercise on PTSD. Anecdotal reports and small-scale studies predominantly inform the available evidence (Roberts et al., 2021). Consequently, caution is warranted when interpreting the findings, and more rigorous research is necessary to establish the efficacy and safety of anaerobic exercise as a therapeutic modality for individuals with PTSD (Arent et al., 2020).

Additionally, the potential drawbacks associated with high-intensity anaerobic exercise for individuals with PTSD must be considered. Engaging in intense anaerobic exercise may inadvertently activate the stress response system and trigger traumatic memories, potentially exacerbating symptoms (Klimek et al., 2018). Therefore, while anaerobic exercise holds promise as a treatment option, further research with robust methodologies is necessary to determine its effectiveness and ascertain appropriate guidelines for its implementation in the context of PTSD.

Flexibility Exercises

Flexibility exercises, such as Pilates, yoga, and stretching, have gained popularity due to their potential to alleviate muscle tension, promote relaxation, and reduce stress and anxiety symptoms (Michailidis et al., 2013). While these exercises offer a mindful and holistic approach to physical fitness and mental well-being, the evidence base regarding their specific effects on PTSD symptoms also remains limited and inconsistent (Pebole et al., 2019).

Some studies have reported positive outcomes, while others found no significant impact or emphasised the need for more extensive, rigorous investigations (Sareen et al., 2022). Furthermore, the underlying physiological and psychological mechanisms through which flexibility exercises exert their benefits on PTSD symptoms are not yet fully understood (Whitworth et al., 2017). Future research should focus on elucidating these mechanisms and exploring potential moderators and mediators of treatment outcomes.

Functional Exercise

Functional exercises, including Tai chi, qigong, dance, high-intensity interval training (HIIT), and CrossFit®, have gained attention for their potential benefits in improving overall fitness and functional capabilities in individuals with anxiety, depression, and PTSD (Claudino et al., 2018; Petz, 2022). These exercises often incorporate elements of balance, coordination, strength, and cardiovascular fitness to enhance both physical and mental well-being (Claudino et al., 2018). However, the evidence regarding the efficacy of functional exercises for PTSD is limited and primarily based on small-scale studies and anecdotal reports (Hegberg et al., 2019).

Additionally, the heterogeneity of functional exercise interventions makes it challenging to draw definitive conclusions about their effectiveness (Thompson et al., 2021). Future research should focus on conducting well-designed randomised controlled trials with larger sample sizes to provide more robust evidence regarding the benefits and limitations of functional exercises for individuals with PTSD.

Personalisation

Despite some positive findings regarding the benefits of physical exercise in treating PTSD, several potential drawbacks warrant consideration (Klimek et al., 2018). Engaging in physical activity can be physically demanding and may trigger traumatic memories and flashbacks in individuals with PTSD, necessitating careful assessment and tailored approaches (Klimek et al., 2018). Healthcare professionals and exercise specialists must be aware of these challenges and develop individualised exercise Programmes that consider the unique needs and preferences of individuals with PTSD (Hegberg et al., 2019).

Moreover, accessibility to physical exercise may present challenges for veterans with physical disabilities, raising concerns about equitable participation and personalised interventions (Björkman & Ekblom, 2022). Efforts should be made to ensure inclusive and accessible exercise environments for all individuals with PTSD, including those with physical limitations (World Health Organization, 2022).

Additionally, conflicting findings in the existing literature, limited sample sizes, and the absence of long-term results hinder the formulation of definitive treatment recommendations (Hegberg et al., 2019). The field would benefit from large-scale, multicentred studies with rigorous methodologies to establish clear guidelines for exercise interventions in PTSD (Van der Kolk et al., 2020) that work for the individual.

Consensus

The existing literature supports the potential benefits of physical exercise, including CrossFit®, in enhancing the well-being and quality of life of individuals with combat-related PTSD (Abel & Benedek, 2019; Forbes et al., 2019; Claudino et al., 2018; Petz, 2021). However, a critical examination of the available studies reveals limitations and gaps in our understanding (Drake et al., 2017). While these findings show promise, it is important to consider the specificity of the evidence and the need for more rigorous research methodologies (Hegberg et al., 2019).

Chapter Aim

In light of the gaps and limitations in the literature regarding the use of specific physical exercise interventions as treatments for PTSD (Asnaani et al., 2014; Whitworth et al., 2017), this chapter examines the effectiveness and feasibility of different exercise modalities in supporting recovery among military veterans. Through interviews with six veterans formally diagnosed with PTSD, the chapter explores their lived experiences and perspectives on exercise as a potential treatment (Shirazipour et al., 2017). By adopting this qualitative approach, the research seeks to shed light on both the benefits and challenges of exercise engagement, as well as the individual variations that influence its role in managing symptoms (Rhodes et al., 2016). In doing so, the findings contribute to the development of evidence-based recommendations designed to optimise well-being and recovery in PTSD (Hegberg et al., 2019).

Importantly, the chapter emphasises the value of capturing the unique perspectives of veterans themselves, whose voices provide depth and nuance often missing in clinical research. In focusing on their accounts, the study situates exercise not only as a therapeutic adjunct but also as a lived practice embedded in daily struggles with PTSD. In this way, the chapter aligns with existing work examining the feasibility of exercise-based interventions in military contexts (Pebole et al., 2019; Diaz & Motta, 2008), highlighting both the potential for positive change and the barriers that may limit access or effectiveness. Ultimately, the discussion underscores the importance of considering exercise as part of a broader therapeutic toolkit for military veterans (Hegberg et al., 2019; Pebole et al., 2019).

Method

Participants and Recruitment

Six military veterans participated in this study, all of whom had received a formal PTSD diagnosis following their service. To ensure relevance, inclusion criteria required that each participant had engaged in physical exercise within the past month, thereby grounding their reflections in recent experiences. Veterans with severe physical health conditions that might prevent meaningful participation were not included. Recruitment was facilitated through Combat Stress, a leading veterans' charity that operates independently from the Ministry of Defence and relies on donations. Their assistance provided access to a diverse group of participants, each able to offer valuable perspectives on the use of exercise as part of PTSD care. Ethical approval was secured, and participants provided informed consent prior to taking part. They were reminded of their right to withdraw at any time, and measures were implemented to protect confidentiality and data security in accordance with best practice (Weathers et al., 1993; Brennan et al., 2016; Arifin, 2018; Peters et al., 2022).

Data Collection Procedure

Semi-structured interviews were used as the primary method of data collection, chosen for their balance of structure and flexibility (Erickson et al., 2015). Participants, all aged 18 or above, were invited to take part either face-to-face or via Zoom, depending on preference. In-person interviews were held in settings selected to promote openness and comfort.

The interviews explored a range of areas including exercise engagement prior to and following PTSD diagnosis, the perceived role of specific exercises in preventing or mitigating episodes, personal accounts of exercise as a coping strategy, and reflections on how exercise compared with psychological therapies or medication in managing symptoms. Veterans were also asked to provide basic demographic information to contextualise their accounts.

Data Analysis

All interviews were transcribed verbatim to preserve accuracy (Mason & Holt, 2012), and the analysis followed Braun and Clarke's (2016) six phases of thematic analysis: familiarisation with the data, generation of codes, searching for themes, reviewing themes, defining and naming themes, and validation. This approach was selected for its accessibility and flexibility, as well as its suitability for inductive, data-driven inquiry (Clarke & Braun, 2013; Braun et al., 2019). The process began with repeated readings of the transcripts to ensure a deep familiarity with the data, followed by systematic coding and the identification of key patterns. These patterns were then refined into broader themes and, where necessary, into sub-themes to capture nuance.

To strengthen the credibility and trustworthiness of the analysis, external validation was undertaken by colleagues with expertise in qualitative research. Following the guidance of Merriam and Grenier (2019), this peer review offered critical feedback and minimised the potential for researcher bias. In presenting the findings, the emphasis is placed on conveying both the common threads across participants' accounts and the diversity of individual experience. In this way, the analysis provides a faithful yet structured representation of how veterans perceive the role of physical exercise in managing PTSD, ensuring that their voices remain central while upholding methodological integrity (Braun & Clarke, 2016; Merriam & Grenier, 2019).

Results

1. Pre-diagnosis Physical Activity and Enjoyment

The first identified theme concerns the importance of Pre-diagnosis physical activity and enjoyment, more importantly, the acknowledgement of the human need to be active (Paluska & Schwenk, 2000; Teixeira et al., 2012). Several participants spoke about their experiences with physical activity prior to their PTSD diagnosis, elaborating on their engagement in a diverse array of sports and exercises.

In describing their exercise, the participants genuinely loved exercise and sports, which probably influenced their choice to join the military. They enjoyed various physical activities like swimming, football, running, and gym workouts, showcasing their diverse interests in staying active. For example, Oscar said:

> Getting fit was essential for joining the military, and my genuine passion for exercise fuelled my dedication. During my military service, I stayed highly active, participating in demanding activities to achieve and maintain peak physical fitness. My love for fitness and discipline greatly influenced my approach to life, instilling a strong work ethic and a determination to tackle challenges.

This was further illustrated, as Bryan commented:

> I remained highly active during my military service, taking part in weekly battalion runs and battalion PT sessions. I often went for solo runs and occasionally used the gym in the evenings. This commitment to fitness and discipline greatly influenced my life, forming a strong work ethic and my capacity to confront challenges directly.

Further highlighting the significant role of physical activity in their lives, participants shared stories vividly showing that it wasn't just about physical fitness. Instead, it became a source of enjoyment and accomplishment deeply ingrained in their core (Patki et al., 2014). Mike said:

> My physical activity levels were consistently high due to my engagement in military exercises integrated into my daily routine. These exercises included fell running, boxing, and dedicated strength training. I also participated in

weekly battalion runs and made frequent visits to the gym in the evenings because I genuinely enjoyed exercising.

This was further illustrated by Sam, who commented:

> Due to my natural love for an active lifestyle and participation in sports, I easily incorporated military-style workouts into my daily routine. My primary focus was on running and rugby, both of which played significant roles. I consistently joined the weekly battalion run and engaged in personal running sessions. Additionally, my passion for exercise motivated me to visit the gym in the evenings, reflecting my genuine commitment to fitness.

The participants talked about how they regularly took part in physical activities since childhood. They mentioned enjoying organised sports and individual exercises that brought them happiness and a sense of purpose. Football, in particular, was a significant passion for them, bringing back memories of teamwork and excitement (Ashdown-Franks et al., 2019). For example, Alex said:

> Before I joined the army, my focus was on football, with fitness taking a back seat. However, military life quickly taught me the importance of being physically ready. The demanding training and fitness routines in the military made it clear how crucial staying in top shape was. Moreover, I noticed that exercise had a positive impact on my mood, helping me achieve a balance between my mental and physical well-being.

Furthermore, Sam also remarked on this sentiment:

> The significance of physical readiness became even clearer when I enlisted in the British military. Engaging in activities like running and strength training introduced me to demanding workouts, reinforcing the substantial benefits of comprehensive fitness routines. Furthermore, I observed that these routines not only improved my physical condition but also positively impacted my mood, helping me to improve my mental health.

In the Chapter, participants experienced relief and a sense of freedom through activities such as running and swimming. These activities provided them with outlets to connect more deeply with their bodies. Engaging in regular running and swimming routines allowed them to take a break from their daily lives, facilitating a balance between their mental and physical well-being (Hegberg et al., 2019).

Before their diagnosis, they had a deep love for physical exercise and experienced the positive emotions it brought. The participants emphasised how exercise significantly improved their overall well-being. For example, Tom said:

> I would have given it my all. Football, my favourite sport, took up a lot of my time, and I made running a daily habit that I truly enjoyed. I also liked to swim when I had the chance. These activities not only boosted my energy but also improved my mood and gave me more self-confidence, helping me face new challenges with resilience and determination.

This became more evident when Ed remarked:

> Football and daily runs brought me happiness and a sense of fulfilment. Through these activities, I felt a clear improvement in my overall well-being, with a boost in my mood, self-confidence, and a greater sense of contentment. Exercise had a significant impact on my life.

Additionally, Cathy agreed:

> I loved staying active and pushed myself to reach my fitness goals. I was fully committed to being as fit as I could be. Cycling and running were big parts of my daily routine, and I enjoyed them immensely. These activities not only boosted my energy but also improved my mood, making me feel better overall.

This illustrates how participants engaged in physical exercise revitalised their energy levels, uplifted their mood, and enhanced their physical fitness. It served as a powerful outlet for stress and provided them with effective coping mechanisms to navigate the challenges they faced (Ashdown-Franks et al., 2019).

Beyond the physical benefits, many participants highlighted how physical activity facilitated other aspects of personal growth and development (Rosenbaum et al., 2015). They spoke passionately about the thrill of competition, the satisfaction of pushing their physical limits, and the profound sense of achievement that accompanied reaching their goals. These experiences nurtured their self-confidence, empowering them to embrace new challenges with resilience and determination (Rosenbaum et al., 2015).

In addition, participants emphasised the social dimension of physical activity. Participation in team sports or training Programmes cultivated a strong sense of belonging and camaraderie with individuals who shared similar interests and goals. For example, Sam said:

> I played rugby and football, and before joining the army, I started running regularly. Once I enlisted, I stuck to daily exercise routines and eventually became a physical training instructor. I genuinely enjoyed exercise, not just for the satisfaction it brought but also for the social connections with my colleagues. I ran every day, played sports, and spent a lot of time in the gym, driven by my love for competition. This boosted my self-confidence and had a positive impact on my overall well-being.

This was underscored when Bryan remarked:

> I began swimming before enlisting, but after basic training, I started to Prioritise gym workouts. This improved my focus, and military life fostered a strong sense of camaraderie. Being part of a team created a profound sense of belonging, motivating me to set clear goals for myself.

The participants shared their deep appreciation for the strong bonds of camaraderie and unwavering support in their experiences. These connections with teammates, coaches, and fellow athletes served as pillars of strength and encouragement. This nurturing environment fostered a passionate pursuit of shared goals (Hegberg et al., 2019).

In these relationships, they shared their determination, which helped maintain their motivation during demanding training sessions (Patki et al., 2014). This commitment led to shared achievements, combining individual successes into collective victories (Björkman & Ekblom, 2022). Participants showed that these connections extended beyond physical activity, forming a supportive network (Rosenbaum et al., 2015). Within this strong sense of camaraderie, the individual journey transitioned from a solo effort to a shared experience, underscoring the close bonds formed through physical engagement. For example, Tony said:

> I remember playing football with my teammates, and the teamwork and motivation we experienced on the field were truly special. It was a bit like the supportive network I later found in the military. These close bonds made every challenge and victory more significant, turning what felt like an individual effort into a shared experience.

Sam further highlighted that these connections extended beyond physical activity by commenting:

> I hold fond memories of playing rugby with my teammates. The strong camaraderie and unity we felt on the field were remarkable, providing motivation and a supportive network that turned what initially seemed like an individual effort into a shared experience. It reminded me of the sense of belonging I later found during my military service.

As participants reflected on their pre-diagnosis physical activities, a strong sense of nostalgia emerged as they shared experiences and mutual encouragement created a positive and motivating environment that further enhanced their enjoyment and commitment to physical activity. For example, Rob said:

> Swimming is like a dependable routine for my body. It's a way of pushing myself, dealing with the cold, covering distances, and challenging my body in a healthy way that reaps both physical and mental benefits. While swimming, I often think back to the good times with friends, and how their encouragement created a positive atmosphere that keeps me motivated and committed to staying active.

This was further illustrated as Bryan commented:

> After 47 years of military service, I've faced various physical and medical challenges due to the demands of such long-term commitment. Nonetheless, I remain committed to staying active through physical activity. It's a constant in my life, reminding me of past experiences and the encouragement I received. This has reinforced my enjoyment and dedication to staying physically active, despite the health issues I've encountered.

Participants recognised the profound impact that exercise had on their mental and emotional well-being during that period. The positive experiences and cherished memories associated with their engagement in physical activity served as a foundation for their understanding of the potential benefits of exercise in managing their PTSD symptoms (Patki et al., 2014) after diagnosis.

In summary, the participants' pre-diagnosis narratives shed light on the myriad benefits of physical activity, encompassing not only joy and fulfilment but also notable improvements in overall well-being. These accounts prompt thoughtful consideration of the potential for structured exercise interventions in the management of PTSD, emphasising the imperative for comprehensive research into underlying mechanisms and their clinical applicability (Ashdown-Franks et al., 2019; Hegberg et al., 2019).

2. Positive Impact of Exercise on PTSD Symptoms

The second theme identified the importance of Positive impact of exercise on PTSD symptoms, more importantly, the acceptance of how physical exercise can have a role in treatment of PTSD being recognised (Ashdown-Franks et al., 2019; Hegberg et al., 2019).

Within this context, it is worth noting that several participants consistently emphasised the profoundly positive impact of regular exercise on alleviating and managing their PTSD symptoms. Their collective accounts converged on the assertion that physical engagement wielded a transformative influence, functioning as a dynamic mechanism to navigate the complex terrain of their psychological challenges and mitigate the often-overwhelming manifestations of PTSD. For example, Ed said:

> engaging in regular exercise, including cold-water swimming and daily cycling, has been a transformative experience for me. Three years ago, I started with limited swimming abilities due to my physical disability, but I've persevered and can now swim a mile, albeit at a slow pace. These activities have played a crucial role in alleviating my PTSD symptoms, helping me navigate the challenges of my condition and providing a positive impact on my mental well-being.

and Cathy was also in agreement and said:

> I found that joining Combat Stress' yoga sessions made a real difference in my life. It helped me shift from feeling stressed to becoming much calmer. This practice was crucial in cultivating a sense of inner peace within me.

By engaging in activities like swimming, cycling, yoga, and running helped them channel their stress and mitigate the likelihood of PTSD episodes. Moreover, the experiences they described as empowering, stress-reducing, and beneficial for their physical and mental well-being (Björkman & Ekblom, 2022). For example, Sam said:

> Exercise, such as swimming, cycling, yoga, and running, gave a sense of empowerment. It's crucial for those dealing with conditions like PTSD and disability, as they can often struggle with self-confidence and independence. Exercise provided a feeling of control and strength.

Tom concurred, stating:

> Using nocturnal running as a strategy has indeed been instrumental in alleviating my symptoms of PTSD. The deliberate shift in the schedule to incorporate nighttime sessions has not only mitigated my symptoms but has also improved my overall sleep quality and well-being.

To further illustrate the calming effect of physical exercise on individuals dealing with distressing memories and intrusive thoughts (Ashdown-Franks et al., 2019; Hegberg et al., 2019), it's noteworthy how engaging in exercise allows them to find a sense of balance and mental clarity. By focusing their energy on the present moment, exercise provides a temporary reprieve from these intrusive thoughts and distressing memories (Adams et al., 2020). For example, Alex said:

> Exercise empowered me, especially during tough times like dealing with PTSD and health problems. It helped me regain my confidence, inner strength and resilience. It also had a calming effect, providing relief from distressing memories and intrusive thoughts. It's clear that physical activity has therapeutic value.

This was further illustrated as Bryan commented, "Participating in physical exercise enabled me to channel my mental energy into daily tasks, effectively countering intrusive thoughts and distressing memories that continued to haunt my mind."

Also, Sam remarked:

> In my experience, physical exercise has a calming effect when dealing with distressing memories and intrusive thoughts. Regular exercise helps me find balance and mental clarity. It allows me to redirect my focus to the present moment, providing relief from those intrusive thoughts and distressing memories. It's like a temporary escape that helps me feel more in control.

Physical exercise helped participants divert their attention from PTSD triggers and anxiety-inducing situations (Hegberg et al., 2019). By focusing on purposeful movement, they found effective relief from overwhelming emotions (Caddick & Smith, 2018). This shift in thinking allowed them to manage their psychological well-being more effectively. For example, Mike said:

> Absolutely, physical exercise has significantly reduced those episodes for me. It has given me a boost in confidence, making me less likely to be afraid or hesitant. With increased confidence, I find it easier to step out the door. Although I still experience episodes almost every morning before going out, even after a year of dedicated swimming, exercise has made a noticeable positive impact.

Sam was also in agreement and said:

> it's reduced, giving me a sense of increased confidence. With higher confidence, I'm less likely to fear something. I feel more confident about going out and engaging with people. However, I still experience episodes of fear and anxiety every morning before heading out, despite engaging in exercise regularly for just over 18 months.

By wholeheartedly engaging in activities that consistently demanded their full attention and engagement, they were skilfully able to engineer precious moments of respite from the otherwise engulfing and overwhelming maelstrom of PTSD symptoms that often sought to dominate their inner landscape (Hegberg et al., 2019). For example, Alex said:

> Yes, I strongly believe exercise plays a significant role in addressing PTSD. I prefer morning runs because I've noticed my symptoms are less severe in the early hours compared to the evenings. Exercise makes me feel liberated, as if I'm taking control of my body and mind. It brings a sense of balance and reaffirms my agency and resilience.

Oscar agreed, "Without a doubt, yes, I strongly believe that exercise is beneficial for dealing with PTSD. I say this because my morning runs help me manage my symptoms, which are more challenging in the evening."

Moreover, exercise was consistently described as not only a means of revitalisation and mental clarity but also as a vitally healthy outlet for managing the burdens of stress, anxiety, and frustration that often beset individuals grappling with the intricacies of PTSD. For example, Sam said:

> engaging in practical exercise in a friendly environment has been a reliable way for me to recharge mentally and find clarity. It also provides a healthy release for the stress, anxiety, and frustration that often accompany my PTSD. Exercise helps me keep these symptoms in check.

and Mike conferred: swimming and cycling are helpful outlets for dealing with my daily stress. They allow me to handle stress proactively and keep it from interfering with my progress. These activities empower me to manage stress without it holding me back.

Additionally, Ed said:

> I've grown to genuinely enjoy exercise, and now, it's an integral part of my daily routine. I've established healthy habits, like going for a swim at the pool, which significantly helps me manage my symptoms. Exercise has become indispensable to my day.

Moreover, participants emphasised how physical activity effectively helped them redirect their negative emotions towards a more productive and positive outlet. For example, Sean said, "Physical activity has undoubtedly become a powerful tool, improving both my physical and mental well-being. It has helped me channel negative emotions in a positive and productive way, making a significant difference in my life."

Additionally, Alex said:

> In my personal experience, this approach has proven to be valuable in handling negative emotions. It effectively allows me to channel these emotions and convert them into a motivating force that drives me towards greater productivity and a more positive outlook on life. This transformation has had a significant and lasting impact on the way I navigate the ups and downs of my daily life.

The release of endorphins, often referred to as the body's natural "feel-good" molecules, during exercise is believed to significantly contribute to overall well-being. This biochemical response may also play a role in reducing the intensity and pervasiveness of PTSD symptoms experienced by individuals (Mikkelsen et al., 2017). However, it is essential to critically assess this connection by considering factors like individual variability and the specific characteristics of exercise. Further research is needed to fully understand the extent of the impact and its clinical implications, as well as the relationship between endorphin release and the alleviation of specific PTSD symptoms (Mikkelsen et al., 2017).

Participants also spoke at length about the profound psychological benefits inherent in regular engagement with exercise. They elaborated on how consistent physical activity acted as a potent catalyst for the cultivation of enhanced self-esteem and self-efficacy, instilling within them a deeply rooted sense of accomplishment and unshakable pride in their remarkable physical achievements. For example, Mike said:

> Rowing in the 5K challenge stresses me, but I see it as a healthy challenge. Despite its difficulty, I can see a clear path to success when I row. Maybe there is something about the simplicity of the task, moving forward toward the finish. The physical benefits from exercise have boosted my self-esteem and confidence because I do hit that line.

and Cathy agreed:

> On the bike, I tackled challenges by pushing myself in intense mountain sessions, even though it was uncomfortable. This helped redirect my thoughts and manage my symptoms. When symptoms flared up, I used physical activity to address both physical and mental challenges, focusing on positive energy use rather than self-criticism. Exercise significantly boosted my self-esteem and self-efficacy.

Through regular exercise, participants harnessed a transformative tool that played a crucial role in building resilience. Their commitment to physical activity also strengthened their mental health against the challenges of PTSD (Caddick & Smith, 2018). Participants noted that the benefits of exercise went beyond physical fitness, enriching various aspects of their lives. For example, Cathy said:

> My commitment to physical activity was vital in building resilience. I started with a Nordic track bike once a week, guided through a training Programme. It began with just three miles weekly, but I grew to love it because it felt like I was enjoying the experience rather than suffering.

and Sam said:

> During the early stages of my diagnosis, incorporating an exercise routine felt challenging. However, as time passed, I came to realise the positive

> impact it had on my well-being. Unfortunately, my physical health eventually declined to a point where even basic walking became too painful to sustain any exercise regime.

Engaging in exercise had a multifaceted impact, extending beyond improving mental well-being. Research supports its positive influence on physical health (Rosenbaum et al., 2015). Participants unanimously felt exercise gave them strength, energy, and readiness to tackle the challenges of PTSD (Rosenbaum et al., 2015). They recognised exercise as a proactive and empowering strategy for managing their condition (Caddick & Smith, 2018). The combination of physical exertion, focused mental engagement, and endorphin release contributed to reducing the frequency and intensity of PTSD episodes (Björkman & Ekblom, 2022).

3. Changes in Behaviour due to Exercise Post-Diagnosis

Theme three identified the importance of Changes in behaviour due to exercise post-diagnosis, more significantly, the awareness of how their PTSD symptoms change due to participating in any form of physical exercise (Stults-Kolehmainen & Sinha, 2014). Some Participants shared how exercise brought about significant changes in their behaviour following their PTSD diagnosis. For example, Sam said, "Diagnosis of my PTSD came after a prolonged period of declining fitness following my active service days. However, I've made significant changes since then. I acquired a peloton bike and now prioritise regular exercise sessions." Bryan agreed by saying:

> Exercising with The Breakfast Club encouraged me to leave the house and made me realise there's more to life outside. Although it's still tough for me to go past those gates, I focus on the positive aspects of these activities.

Participants emphasised the significant change they underwent, both physically and mentally, thanks to their commitment to regular exercise routines. This transformation highlighted the substantial impact of their efforts, something supported by research (Mikkelsen et al., 2017).

Participants notably transformed their approach to physical activity by adopting structured exercise routines. This change had significant implications for their well-being and daily routines. For example, Cathy said:

> I swim a mile every morning, aiming to complete it in around 50 minutes, five times a week. In the afternoon, I cycle 8 to 10 miles, also five times a week. This structured exercise routine has become a significant part of my daily life, positively impacting my well-being and daily routines.

This was further acknowledged by Rob who said:

> Swimming has become my sanctuary, allowing me to channel anxiety and overcome negative thoughts. The rhythm of strokes creates a calming cadence that propels me towards a more positive state of mind.

By incorporating activities like swimming, cycling, and running into their daily lives, they illustrated how important it is in making exercise a priority (Oppizzi & Umberger, 2018). Furthermore, by adhering to a routine, they experienced a sense of discipline and consistency that positively influenced their overall well-being (Ley et al., 2018).

Engaging in exercise brought significant changes in participants' physical abilities. Many started with short swimming distances or faced challenges in cycling initially. Over time, they witnessed tangible improvements in their performance and endurance, thanks to dedication and perseverance. This highlighted their inherent potential for growth through physical engagement. For example, Ed said:

> I started my exercise routine in the morning but faced problems. I shifted it to nighttime when family commitments allowed. This change helped me get more from my routine, and I've seen improvements in my performance and endurance. It highlights the potential for growth through exercise and has also helped my mental health.

This was agreed by Steve:

> I've come to enjoy my morning exercise routine. My military background instilled discipline, helping me set goals and achieve milestones. This improved my performance and endurance, providing a sense of purpose and accomplishment, benefiting my physical and mental well-being.

Participants credited these changes to their determination, perseverance, and commitment to their exercise routines. They found satisfaction in pushing their physical boundaries and achieving personal goals, despite the challenges posed by their PTSD or physical disabilities (Shirazipour et al., 2017).

Participants also noted a shift in their mindset and attitude towards physical activity. Through consistent engagement, they developed a more positive view of exercise (Rosenbaum et al., 2015). This transformation involved seeing physical activity not just as exertion but as a tool for self-care, nurturing their mental and emotional well-being (Ley et al., 2018). For example, Bryan said:

> I tried to push myself harder on days when I thought I might have an off day. If things were difficult the night before due to PTSD or other challenges, I aimed to channel some of that aggression and anger through exercise. It helped me normalize the rest of my day, and I can't relate it to anything else.

Tom agreed by saying,

> I have changed how I see physical activity. It's no longer just about physical exertion; it's become a powerful tool for self-care, helping me protect and nurture my mental and emotional well-being.

Furthermore, participants realised that exercise provided strong motivation, driving them to push their limits and achieve feats of physical and mental resilience. For example, Ed said, "On a personal level, exercise served as a strong motivation. It went beyond just physical exertion and became a driving force in my journey. Each workout and every effort renewed my dedication to my physical and mental health, pushing my limits and building resilience".

and Sam said:

> I personally found exercise to be a powerful source of motivation. It went beyond just physical activity and became a driving force in my life. Every step and every weight lifted filled me with energy, purpose and built my mental resilience. It was a constant reminder of my dedication and commitment to my own well-being.

Exercise held a significant and enduring purpose in their daily routines, seamlessly blending into their lives. This consistent engagement provided structure and served as a guiding force in their pursuit of overall well-being (Whitworth & Ciccolo, 2016). It was not only a routine but also a source of motivation, leading them towards achieving holistic health and vitality (Whitworth & Ciccolo, 2016).

In addition to these changes, participants spoke about the impact of exercise on their overall behaviour and lifestyle. They noticed that engaging in regular physical activity helped them adopt healthier habits and make positive choices in other areas of their lives. For example, Tom said:

> A regular exercise routine motivated me to start each day with structure and productivity. I wake up, make my bed, empty the dishwasher, get some coffee, and then head to my exercise routine. I think this routine helps me by improving not only my physical well-being but also overall organization and efficiency.

and Oscar said:

> Incorporating regular training and exercise has become a significant part of my daily routine. It has brought anticipation and eagerness into my life, which was lacking before. This change has also impacted my overall behaviour and lifestyle positively.

Exercise became a catalyst, driving personal growth and promoting a health-conscious lifestyle. This progression triggered a chain of positive effects, ultimately improving their overall mental well-being and resilience (Mikkelsen et al., 2017; Whitworth et al., 2017).

Participants acknowledged that engaging in exercise necessitated a blend of earnest effort, steadfast commitment, and unwavering determination. These traits, they realised, possessed a remarkable transferability that seamlessly extended well beyond the realm of their exercise routines. For Example, Sam said:

> I've developed a strong passion for exercise, and I genuinely can't imagine my day without it. These healthy habits have seamlessly become a part of my daily routine. I eagerly prepare, head out the door, hop into my car, and head to the pool for a revitalising swim.

and the same sentiment was experienced by Tom,

> I've developed a deep appreciation for exercise, seamlessly integrating it into my daily routine. It's become a vital part of my well-being, adding energy and direction to each moment, bringing about a positive transformation in my life.

The discipline and perseverance honed through exercise proved to be a wellspring of empowerment, flowing into diverse facets of their lives. This spill-over effect played a pivotal role in guiding them through the intricate challenges entwined with their PTSD. Additionally, these attributes acted as catalysts for fostering personal growth and cultivating resilience, as illuminated by scholarly research (Fetzner & Asmundson, 2015; Rosenbaum et al., 2015).

Overall, participants recognised the profound changes in their behaviour that resulted from incorporating exercise into their lives (Caddick & Smith, 2018). They developed structured routines, observed improvements in physical capabilities, adopted positive mindsets, and made healthier choices (Hegberg et al., 2019). Exercise became a catalyst for personal growth, promoting discipline, perseverance, and resilience (Rosenbaum et al., 2015).

4. Exercise Compared to Other Treatments

The fourth theme identified the importance of Exercise compared to other treatments, more significantly, participants acknowledged how exercise contrasts from other tried and tested traditional treatment methods for PTSD (Björkman & Ekblom, 2022; Lee et al., 2022). Participants provided insights into their perceptions of exercise compared to other treatments for PTSD. For example, Sam said:

> CBT hasn't worked well for me. Exercise, along with integrative psychotherapy, has been my main support. When I started, I didn't understand my emotions. Exercise helps me regain control, reduce pain, and sleep better, which CBT and other treatments didn't do.

Furthermore, Cathy said:

> Cognitive Behavioural Therapy didn't work well for me, but I found benefits in integrative psychotherapy and exercise. Initially, I lacked emotional insight. Unlike CBT, exercise helps me regain emotional control, manage pain, and improve my sleep.

Oscar concurs:

> CBT didn't work well for me, but integrative psychotherapy and exercise have been pivotal in my transformation. Initially, I struggled with emotions, but exercise has helped me regain control and manage discomfort, leading to better sleep compared to CBT and other therapies.

Participants underscored exercise's distinct effectiveness in managing their symptoms, setting it apart from psychological techniques and medications. It injected vitality and transformative power into their holistic well-being journey, complementing traditional methods (Oppizzi & Umberger, 2018).

As shown above, participants in this Chapter showed reservations about Cognitive-Behavioural Therapy (CBT) and its suitability for their needs. They described a preference for alternative therapeutic modalities such as integrative psychotherapy. For example, Sam said:

> While I did try mindfulness and CBT, I found that these psychological approaches didn't have the same positive impact. However, through exercise, I discovered a strong sense of worthiness and well-being that is highly valuable to me and well worth pursuing.

and Bryan agrees by saying, "When it comes to the psychological aspect, like CBT, it doesn't really connect with me. Personally, I've found that exercise is the most effective approach for dealing with and managing my PTSD symptoms." They felt that CBT did not adequately address their emotional experiences or provide them with a deeper understanding of their emotions. Instead, they found that exercise, with its physical and mental benefits, offered a more holistic and fulfilling approach to their healing journey (Shirazipour et al., 2017; Whitworth et al., 2017).

Participants acknowledged that exercise helped them develop a better connection with their bodies and emotions. Engaging in physical activity enabled them to live in the present moment, fostering a sense of mindfulness and self-awareness. For example, Sam said:

> I've personally explored both CBT and mindfulness techniques, even confronting my triggers along the way. Yet, despite my dedication to these approaches, I've come to realise that they haven't had the same impact on reducing my daily PTSD episodes as engaging in physical exercise has.

and Alex remarks:

> During the COVID-19 pandemic, I had to adapt to life without medication. To my surprise, this change taught me how to manage daily tasks, control my emotions, and effectively handle my PTSD symptoms. This newfound empowerment allowed me to identify and meet my personal needs, eliminating the need for medication. Engaging in physical exercise was a key factor in alleviating my PTSD symptoms.

They held a profound appreciation for the mind-body connection fostered by exercise. This connection enabled them to effectively process their emotions, alleviate stress, and attain a more profound self-awareness. Their experiences underscored the holistic benefits of physical activity (Ashdown-Franks et al., 2019).

Furthermore, participants engaged in introspection regarding the efficacy of exercise as compared to medication in their journeys. They recognised the unique advantages of physical activity in managing their symptoms and promoting overall well-being. For example, Alex said:

> In my experience, a combination of exercise and medication has proven most effective. Exercise significantly enhances my mood and stress management, while I continue to take medication at night to improve my sleep. This approach acknowledges the importance of medication for sleep and the stress management benefits of exercise.

Ed concurred, stating:

> I've learned to appreciate the importance of both my prescribed medication and physical exercise. Combining these two approaches allows me to use medication for better sleep and exercise to alleviate my anxiety and stress.

Participants have differing views on medication. Some find it helpful, while others worry about side effects. This shows a preference for alternative approaches to manage their condition. For example, Mike said:

> Looking back on my journey, I've found that psychological medical treatments have produced positive results. The techniques I've learned have become essential parts of my routine, consistently helping me maintain my well-being and manage my symptoms.

Tom agreed:

> I've learned that a combination of medication and exercise is crucial in managing the effects of my PTSD, along with the associated experiences of depression and anxiety that I suffer from. This combined approach has been essential for maintaining my well-being and quality of life.

Participants valued exercise for its holistic advantages, acknowledging its positive influence on physical health and overall well-being (Stults-Kolehmainen & Sinha, 2014). They also recognised exercise as a source of control and empowerment, distinguishing it from concerns about medications that might dampen emotions. Exercise emerged as an effective tool for managing and alleviating PTSD symptoms in their view (Ashdown-Franks et al., 2019; Hegberg et al., 2019).

In the broader context, participants viewed exercise as a valuable and effective treatment, surpassing psychological techniques and medications (Hegberg et al., 2019). They appreciated exercise's holistic benefits, its impact on mind-body connection, and the empowerment it offered (Whitworth et al., 2017). While acknowledging other treatment benefits, participants found exercise uniquely suited to their needs and contributing to their overall well-being (Rosenbaum et al., 2015).

In summary, the participants' experiences and perspectives shed light on the role of physical exercise in addressing PTSD among military veterans. These insights align with existing research findings (Björkman & Ekblom, 2022; Lee et al., 2022). The interviews underscored the importance of physical activity both before and after diagnosis, highlighting the genuine enjoyment participants found in it (Paluska & Schwenk, 2000; Teixeira et al., 2012).

They emphasised exercise's substantial positive influence on managing PTSD symptoms, fostering behavioural changes through regular physical activity, and its notable effectiveness when compared to other treatments (Ashdown-Franks et al., 2019; Hegberg et al., 2019). These themes collectively illustrate the significant potential of physical exercise as a therapeutic tool for enhancing the well-being of military veterans grappling with PTSD, offering holistic benefits encompassing their physical, mental, and emotional dimensions.

Chapter Discussion

PTSD presents a significant mental health challenge for military veterans, emphasising the need for effective symptom management strategies. This Chapter examined the experiences and perspectives of military veterans with PTSD, focusing on the role of physical exercise in alleviating their symptoms (Hegberg et al., 2019; Herbert et al., 2020). By analysing interviews with six participants, four key themes emerged:

Pre-Diagnosis Physical Activity and Enjoyment

Before their PTSD diagnosis, physical activity held a significant role in the lives of the participants, aligning with the expectations of British military combat soldiers to engage in physical exercise and maintain fitness (Paluska & Schwenk, 2000; Teixeira et al., 2012). They actively participated in various sports and exercises, deriving deep satisfaction, a sense of accomplishment, and enjoyment from these pursuits (Patki et al., 2014). Starting at a young age, physical exercise became an integral part of their daily routines, offering not only physical fitness but also a source of pleasure and purpose (Rosenbaum et al., 2015). These findings are consistent with prior research emphasising the positive influence of physical activity on overall well-being and mental health (Ashdown-Franks et al., 2019; Hegberg et al., 2019).

Positive Impact of Exercise on PTSD Symptoms

The therapeutic benefits of exercise for managing PTSD symptoms were evident (Ashdown-Franks et al., 2019; Hegberg et al., 2019). Participants reported that activities like swimming, cycling, yoga, and running helped them cope with stress, reduce the likelihood of PTSD episodes, and experience a sense of release (Adams et al., 2020). Exercise provided them with a way to temporarily escape intrusive thoughts and distressing memories (Björkman & Ekblom, 2022). Moreover, exercise acted as a healthy outlet for stress, anxiety, and frustration, with the release of endorphins contributing to a decrease in the frequency and intensity of PTSD episodes. These findings align with the broader literature emphasising the positive impact of exercise on mental health and its potential as an adjunctive treatment for PTSD (Björkman & Ekblom, 2022; Lee et al., 2022).

Changes in Behaviour Due to Exercise Post-Diagnosis

Engaging in regular exercise routines led to significant behaviour changes post-diagnosis (Stults-Kolehmainen & Sinha, 2014). Participants developed structured exercise routines, witnessed improvements in physical capabilities, embraced positive mindsets, and made healthier choices. Exercise served as a catalyst for personal growth, discipline, perseverance, and resilience (Mikkelsen et al., 2017). Participants recognised exercise as a means of self-care, vital for maintaining their mental and emotional well-being (Caddick & Smith, 2018). These findings support previous research highlighting the transformative impact of exercise on behaviour and lifestyle changes (Hegberg et al., 2019; Whitworth et al., 2017).

Exercise Compared to Other Treatments

Participants' perceptions of exercise compared to traditional treatment approaches for PTSD, such as CBT and medications, revealed unique benefits (Björkman & Ekblom, 2022; Lee et al., 2022). Some participants expressed reservations about the effectiveness of CBT and found exercise to be a more holistic and fulfilling approach to their healing journey (Oppizzi & Umberger, 2018). They valued the mind-body connection that exercise facilitated and appreciated its empowering nature. Participants acknowledged that exercise provided them with a sense of control and allowed them to actively participate in their healing process (Oppizzi & Umberger, 2018). These findings suggest that exercise has a distinct role to play in the treatment of PTSD and may complement existing therapies (Ashdown-Franks et al., 2019; Hegberg et al., 2019).

Considerations

This chapter is not a definitive answer as to the questions of whether exercise will work for all PTSD sufferers. Nor does this chapter, and it's limited sample size, help us understand which type of exercise is most effective for those that it does help. However, this Chapter provides essential insights into the role of physical exercise in managing PTSD symptoms among military veterans who were formally into exercise prior to joining the military and prior to diagnosis.

This means that there is a self-selection criteria at play with this sample. It cannot say that those unengaged or bothered by exercise will benefit from it as a treatment for PTSD. However, because members of the armed services must pass physical fitness tests, it is reasonable to suggest that this self-selection criteria exists prior to joining the military and not after receiving PTSD, and therefore it lends more prima facie validity to the usefulness of exercise among veterans.

Participants' accounts of pre-diagnosis physical activity underscore the significance of exercise in their lives and its potential as a therapeutic tool (Whitworth et al., 2017). Engaging in physical exercise was linked to enjoyment, fulfilment, and a profound sense of accomplishment. Additionally, exercise had a positive impact on overall well-being, including increased energy levels, improved mood, and enhanced physical fitness. Participants also experienced positive behaviour changes, including structured routines, improved capabilities, and healthier habits.

The therapeutic benefits of exercise for managing PTSD symptoms were evident in a multitude of ways with the participants' stated experiences. Engaging in physical activity provided them with a sense of release, a coping mechanism for their symptoms, and a temporary escape from intrusive thoughts and distressing memories (Stults-Kolehmainen & Sinha, 2014). Exercise was described as a healthy outlet for stress, anxiety, and frustration, with endorphin release contributing to reduced PTSD episode frequency and intensity. Furthermore, exercise was associated with personal growth, discipline, perseverance, and resilience (Hegberg et al., 2019), empowering participants to actively participate in their healing process and gain control over their bodies and minds.

Participants' preference for exercise over traditional treatments also suggests that exercise offers unique benefits in managing PTSD symptoms (Paluska & Schwenk, 2000). While some expressed reservations about traditional approaches like CBT and medications, they found exercise to be a holistic and empowering approach whether combined with other treatment options or not. Exercise was seen as a means of self-care, crucial for maintaining mental and emotional well-being. This highlights exercise's potential as a valuable complement to existing therapies (Paluska & Schwenk, 2000; Teixeira et al., 2012).

Equally as important, none of the participants expressed negative effects of exercise on their PTSD. Again, the small sample size rules out generalisability, but it is at least evidence of a trend among PTSD sufferers who valued exercise prior to their trauma (Hegberg et al., 2019). The limited number of participants also restricts our capacity to draw wide-reaching conclusions or to make definitive recommendations (Klimek et al., 2018) about which type of exercise is most effective for these participants.

Furthermore, it is worth noting that our recruitment process relied solely on Combat Stress, a charitable organisation dedicated to supporting veterans dealing with PTSD. This approach could potentially introduce another form of selection bias into our Chapter, as our participants are individuals who are actively seeking assistance and motivated to address their PTSD symptoms. Consequently, the sample may not fully represent the broader population of even physically active individuals with PTSD (Murphy et al., 2019; Williamson et al., 2019). Additionally, the absence of a control group in our Chapter prevents direct comparisons with other treatment approaches or a no-intervention condition (McArdle et al., 2010; Patel et al., 2017).

These limitations should be carefully considered when interpreting our Chapter's findings and underscore the necessity for future research with more substantial and diverse participant samples, as well as controlled Chapter designs. Such efforts are essential to establish more robust evidence and facilitate the generalisation of our findings to broader populations (Hegberg et al., 2019). For now, what it does suggest is that for those who enjoyed exercise before their diagnosis, and for those motivated to help reduce their suffering, exercise was a valuable tool in their arsenal.

Chapter Conclusion

In summary, this chapter contributes to the growing body of evidence supporting the therapeutic benefits of physical exercise in alleviating PTSD symptoms among military veterans. It's important to acknowledge that this research is based on a small sample of six participants, necessitating further investigation on a larger scale to either corroborate or challenge these findings.

To facilitate this transition to the next phase of our research, the upcoming Chapter will involve the distribution of a quantitative online survey questionnaire to a wider spectrum of military veterans with PTSD. This broader investigation aims to determine whether the positive effects of physical exercise observed in our initial six participants hold true for a more extensive veteran community.

The results continue to underscore the positive impact of exercise on overall well-being, symptom management, and behaviour change. The integration of exercise into treatment plans offers a holistic approach to support veterans with PTSD, allowing us to customise exercise regimes according to individual preferences and goals. This chapter sets the stage for further exploration and validation of these findings in the upcoming research.

References

Abel, K., & Benedek, D. M. (2019). Military service, trauma, and mental health in veterans. In D. M. Benedek & G. H. Wynn (Eds.), *Complementary and integrative treatments in psychiatry*. American Psychiatric Association Publishing.

Adams, J., Smith, L., & Thomas, E. (2020). Physical activity, affect regulation, and post-traumatic stress: A narrative review. *Journal of Mental Health and Physical Activity, 18*.

Adler, A. B., & Sipos, M. L. (2018). The mental health of soldiers. In L. W. Roberts (Ed.), *Military and veteran mental health*. Springer.

Andreasen, N. C. (2010). *Posttraumatic stress disorder: A history and a critique*. American Psychiatric Publishing.

Arent, S. M., Walker, A. J., & Gleim, A. J. (2020). Resistance training and mental health: Current perspectives. *Sports Medicine, 50*.

Arifin, W. N. (2018). Ethical considerations in qualitative research. *International Journal of Care Scholars, 1*(2).

Armour, C., McBride, O., Shevlin, M., & Carragher, N. (2015). Re-experiencing, avoidance, and hyperarousal in PTSD: A review of latent structure. *Behavioural and Cognitive Psychotherapy, 43*(2).

Armour, C., Müllerová, J., & Elhai, J. D. (2016). A systematic literature review of PTSD's latent structure. *Clinical Psychology Review, 44*.

Ashdown-Franks, G., Firth, J., Carney, R., Carvalho, A. F., Hallgren, M., Koyanagi, A., … Stubbs, B. (2019). Exercise as medicine for mental health. *Current Sports Medicine Reports, 18*(6).

Asnaani, A., McLean, C. P., & Foa, E. B. (2014). Updating PTSD treatment research: From efficacy to implementation. *Clinical Psychology: Science and Practice, 21*(3).

Björkman, A., & Ekblom, Ö. (2022). Exercise, stress regulation, and trauma-related symptoms: Mechanisms and applications. *Scandinavian Journal of Medicine & Science in Sports, 32*(2).

Braun, V., & Clarke, V. (2016). (Mis)conceptualising themes, thematic analysis, and other problems with Braun and Clarke (2006). *International Journal of Social Research Methodology, 19*(6).

Braun, V., Clarke, V., & Weate, P. (2019). Using thematic analysis in sport and exercise research. In B. Smith & A. C. Sparkes (Eds.), *Routledge handbook of qualitative research in sport and exercise* (2nd ed.). Routledge.

Brennan, C., Rhodes, R. E., & Murray, T. (2016). Qualitative methods in exercise psychology. *Qualitative Research in Sport, Exercise and Health, 8*(4).

Caddick, N., & Smith, B. (2018). Exercise as a social practice for veterans with PTSD. *Qualitative Research in Sport, Exercise and Health, 10*(1).

Clarke, V., & Braun, V. (2013). Teaching thematic analysis. *The Psychologist, 26*(2).

Claudino, J. G., Gabbett, T. J., Bourgeois, F., Souza, H. S., Miranda, R. C., Mezêncio, B., et al. (2018). CrossFit overview: Systematic review and meta-analysis. *Sports Medicine – Open, 4*(11).

Diaz, A., & Motta, R. (2008). The effects of an aerobic exercise programme on PTSD symptoms. *International Journal of Emergency Mental Health, 10*(1).

Drake, N. B., Smeed, J., Carper, M. J., & Crawford, D. A. (2017). Effects of CrossFit on health. *Journal of Strength and Conditioning Research, 31*(11).

Erickson, K. I., Hillman, C., & Kramer, A. F. (2015). Physical activity, brain, and cognition. *Current Opinion in Behavioral Sciences, 4.*

Fetzner, M. G., & Asmundson, G. J. G. (2015). Aerobic exercise for PTSD: A review. *Annals of the New York Academy of Sciences, 1341*(1).

Forbes, D., Bisson, J. I., Monson, C. M., & Berliner, L. (2019). *Effective treatments for PTSD* (3rd ed.). Guilford Press.

Hegberg, N. J., Hayes, J. P., & Hayes, S. M. (2019). Exercise intervention in PTSD: A narrative review. *CNS Neuroscience & Therapeutics, 25*(10).

Herbert, C., Meixner, F., Wiebking, C., & Gilg, V. (2020). Regular exercise and mental health. *Psychology & Health, 35*(11).

Klimek, L., Bergmann, K.-C., & Biedermann, T. (2018). High-intensity training considerations in mental health. *European Archives of Psychiatry and Clinical Neuroscience, 268*(4).

Kurowski, A., Parker, S., & Taylor, J. (2017). Aerobic training dose and PTSD symptoms. *Psychiatry Research, 256.*

Lee, D. J., Schnitzlein, C. W., Wolf, J. P., Vythilingam, M., & Rasmusson, A. M. (2022). Psychotherapy versus pharmacotherapy for PTSD: A review. *Current Psychiatry Reports, 24.*

Ley, C., Rato Barrio, M., & Koch, A. (2018). *Sport and physical activity for mental health.* Springer.

Livingston, W. S., Boyda, D., & Macdonald, S. (2021). PTSD: Diagnostic issues and updates. *BJPsych Advances, 27*(5).

Mason, J., & Holt, R. (2012). *Qualitative researching* (3rd ed.). Sage.

McArdle, W. D., Katch, F. I., & Katch, V. L. (2010). *Exercise physiology: Nutrition, energy, and human performance* (7th ed.). Lippincott Williams & Wilkins.

Merriam, S. B., & Grenier, R. S. (2019). *Qualitative research in practice* (2nd ed.). Jossey-Bass.

Michailidis, Y., Fatouros, I. G., & Primpa, E. (2013). Plyometrics and flexibility: Effects on performance. *Journal of Strength and Conditioning Research, 27*(12).
Mikkelsen, K., Stojanovska, L., Polenakovic, M., Bosevski, M., & Apostolopoulos, V. (2017). Exercise and mental health: Biological mechanisms. *Brain, Behavior, and Immunity, 61.*
Murphy, D., Spencer-Henshall, R., & Turgoose, D. (2019). Help-seeking in UK veterans with PTSD. *European Journal of Psychotraumatology, 10*(1).
O'Donovan, G., Blazevich, A. J., & Boreham, C. (2010). The ABC of prescribing exercise. *British Journal of Sports Medicine, 44*(12).
Oppizzi, L. M., & Umberger, R. (2018). Exercise variables in PTSD: A scoping review. *Military Medicine, 183*(3–4).
Paluska, S. A., & Schwenk, T. L. (2000). Physical activity and mental health. *Sports Medicine, 29*(3).
Patel, H., Alkhawam, H., Madanieh, R., Shah, N., Kosmas, C. E., & Vittorio, T. J. (2017). Aerobic vs. anaerobic exercise on cardiovascular health. *World. Journal of Cardiology, 9*(2).
Patki, G., Solanki, N., Atrooz, F., Allam, F., & Salim, S. (2014). Depression, anxiety, and exercise: A review. *Neuroscience & Biobehavioural Reviews, 43.*
Pebole, M. M., Hall, K. S., & Morey, M. C. (2019). Exercise feasibility in military populations with PTSD. *Military Medicine, 184*(11–12).
Peters, M. D. J., Godfrey, C., McInerney, P., … (2022). Ethical and practical considerations in qualitative interviewing. *International Journal of Qualitative Methods, 21.*
Petz, M. R. (2021). Examining the contributions of grit, mental toughness, and conscientiousness to athletic performance (Doctoral dissertation). Capella University.
Petz, M. R. (2022). Mental toughness and performance in functional fitness. *International Journal of Sports Psychology, 53*(4).
Rhodes, R. E., Janssen, I., Bredin, S. S. D., Warburton, D. E. R., & Bauman, A. (2016). Physical activity: Health impact and promotion. *Applied Physiology, Nutrition, and Metabolism, 42*(3).
Roberts, A. L., Chan, L., & Gardner, B. (2021). Resistance training and PTSD symptoms: A pilot study. *Psychiatry Research, 300.*
Rosenbaum, S., Sherrington, C., & Tiedemann, A. (2015). Exercise and mental health: Translating evidence. *American Journal of Lifestyle Medicine, 9*(6).
Sareen, J., Jones, S., & Stein, M. B. (2022). Mind–body interventions for trauma. *Depression and Anxiety, 39*(4).
Shirazipour, C. H., Hains, K., Balchin, R., & Latimer-Cheung, A. E. (2017). The role of physical activity in recovery from PTSD: Veterans' perspectives. *Qualitative Health Research, 27*(12).
Smith, A., Jones, B., & Brown, C. (2020). Aerobic exercise dose and PTSD outcomes: Mixed findings. *Journal of Affective Disorders, 277.*

Smith, P., & Merwin, R. (2021). Resistance training for anxiety-related disorders. *Current Psychiatry Reports, 23*(6).

Stonerock, G. L., Hoffman, B. M., Smith, P. J., & Blumenthal, J. A. (2015). Exercise dose in mental health. *Psychiatric Clinics of North America, 38*(4).

Stults-Kolehmainen, M. A., & Sinha, R. (2014). The effects of stress on physical activity and exercise. *Sports Medicine, 44*(1).

Teixeira, P. J., Carraca, E. V., Markland, D., Silva, M. N., & Ryan, R. M. (2012). Exercise, self-determination, and behaviour change. *International Journal of Behavioural Nutrition and Physical Activity, 9.*

Thompson, W. R., Sallis, R., & Joy, E. (2021). Exercise is medicine: From idea to implementation. *Current Sports Medicine Reports, 20*(9).

Van der Kolk, B., Hodgdon, H., & Gapen, M. (2020). Exercise, yoga, and trauma: Mechanisms and outcomes. *European Journal of Psychotraumatology, 11*(1).

Weathers, F. W., Litz, B. T., Herman, D. S., Huska, J. A., & Keane, T. M. (1993). The PTSD Checklist (PCL): Reliability, validity, and diagnostic utility. Paper presented at the Annual Convention of the International Society for Traumatic Stress Studies, San Antonio, TX.

Whitworth, J. W., & Ciccolo, J. T. (2016). Exercise and PTSD: A systematic review. *American Journal of Lifestyle Medicine, 10*(5).

Whitworth, J. W., Craft, L. L., Dunsiger, S. I., & Ciccolo, J. T. (2017). Aerobic, resistance, and mind–body exercise for PTSD. *Psychological Trauma: Theory, Research, Practice, and Policy, 9*(1).

Whitworth, J. W., Sandoval, R. S., & Lanni, L. (2019). Resistance training for symptoms of PTSD: Preliminary evidence. *Mental Health and Physical Activity, 16.*

Williamson, V., Murphy, D., Phelps, A., Forbes, D., & Greenberg, N. (2019). Help-seeking for PTSD in veterans: Barriers and facilitators. *European Journal of Psychotraumatology, 10*(1).

World Health Organization. (2022). *Guidelines on physical activity and sedentary behaviour*. World Health Organization.

CHAPTER 6

Examining PTSD and Exercise in Military Veterans

Throughout history, soldiers have endured challenges and lasting consequences of their service, with military personnel, including those from the British military, facing deployments to various theatres of operation, such as the conflict in Iraq. These deployments often expose them to traumatic events, contributing to a significant rise in the prevalence of Post-Traumatic Stress Disorder (PTSD) among military veterans (Caddick & Smith, 2014; Hegberg et al., 2019). PTSD poses a formidable challenge for military veterans, and conventional prescribed treatments have yielded mixed results, often due to the severity of symptoms or the prolonged duration of treatment (Björkman & Ekblom, 2022).

Given the substantial impact of PTSD on both serving personnel and military veterans following traumatic battlefield experiences (Abeyasinghe et al., 2012), researchers are intensifying their efforts to comprehend the difficulties of PTSD symptomology and develop more effective treatments (Cukor et al., 2010; Walker et al., 2016). Battlefield experiences, characterised by prolonged exposure to threats and the loss of life, necessitate a comprehensive understanding of the root causes of PTSD and its specific trauma associations (Yehuda et al., 2014).

Contemporary research on PTSD and its treatments reveals the complex reality of managing PTSD symptoms amongst military veterans (Cloitre, 2009; Thompson-Hollands et al., 2021). Both pharmacological and psychological interventions have displayed varying levels of

J. Alder, *Military Men, Physical Exercise, and Post-Traumatic Stress Disorder*, Palgrave Studies in Masculinity, Sport and Exercise,
https://doi.org/10.1007/978-3-032-08957-1_6

effectiveness, but their universal applicability is uncertain, as indicated by Hegberg et al., 2019 in Chap. 4. This highlights the importance of recognising the substantial variability in symptoms among individuals with PTSD, emphasising the need for a more tailored and holistic approach, especially for veterans (Bisson et al., 2020; Libby et al., 2012).

Furthermore, considering the mixed results from conventional prescribed treatments (Bjorkman & Ekblom, 2022), it becomes crucial to conduct a comprehensive evaluation of alternative holistic options, particularly with military veterans. This research can illuminate the efficacy of alternatives treatments relative to established treatments (Wahbeh et al., 2014). A thorough exploration of these factors is pivotal in optimising care for individuals grappling with PTSD.

There has been a growing interest in exploring the potential of physical exercise as a treatment for military veterans grappling with PTSD. This chapter delves into the diverse field of physical exercises to assess their viability as therapeutic interventions for veterans with PTSD. Here, physical exercise is universally recognised as a cornerstone of cardiovascular fitness and overall well-being (McArdle et al., 2010; Patel et al., 2017).

Furthermore, Hegberg et al. (2019) emphasise the versatility of physical exercise, spanning across various forms, including aerobic exercises (e.g., walking, running, and swimming), anaerobic activities (e.g., weightlifting and resistance training), flexibility exercises (e.g., Pilates and yoga), and functional exercises (e.g., Tai chi, qigong, dance, HIIT, and CrossFit®). Each of these forms of physical exercise brings unique benefits to both physical and mental health (Papazoglou & Andersen, 2014; Hegberg et al., 2019).

For instance, aerobic exercises have shown promise in improving cardiovascular health and mitigating PTSD symptoms such as anxiety, depression, hyperarousal, and sleep disturbances (Hegberg et al., 2019). On the other hand, anaerobic exercises contribute to enhanced muscle strength and power, reduction in anger, avoidance behaviours, and emotional stress cues (Wahbeh et al., 2014). At the same time, flexibility exercises play a crucial role in alleviating muscle tension, calming and relaxation, and reducing symptoms of stress and anxiety (Michailidis et al., 2013). Finally, functional exercises, including activities like Tai chi, qigong, dance, HIIT, and CrossFit®, not only enhance overall fitness and functional capacity but also contribute to increased self-confidence and decreased symptoms of anxiety, depression, and avoidance behaviours (Claudino et al., 2018; Petz, 2021).

Despite the compelling evidence regarding the therapeutic benefits of physical exercise in addressing PTSD, Hegberg et al. (2019) caution against potential challenges. Physical exercise, while beneficial, can also be physically demanding, potentially triggering traumatic memories and flashbacks for individuals with PTSD (Claudino et al., 2018). Moreover, accessibility to physical exercise may pose limitations, particularly for veterans with physical disabilities (Björkman & Ekblom, 2022). Additionally, existing literature on this topic presents conflicting findings, partly due to small sample sizes and a lack of long-term results, which restrict the formulation of concrete treatment recommendations. Hence, there is a need for further research into the role of physical exercise as a potential treatment modality for military veterans grappling with PTSD (Hegberg et al., 2019).

One area within the domain of physical exercise that warrants further examination is CrossFit®, due to its multifaceted nature. Chapter 7 employs an autoethnographic approach to assess CrossFit® as a potential treatment method for PTSD, providing an overview of the protagonist's journey and its direct impact on PTSD symptom management. Drawing from the fundamental principles of autonomy, competence, and relatedness within the context of Self-Determination Theory (SDT) (Deci & Ryan, 1985; Edmunds et al., 2006), this chapter explored the protagonist's experience.

Additionally, during pandemic-induced lockdowns, the protagonist's decision to engage with CrossFit® symbolised their reassertion of personal agency, a pivotal aspect of PTSD treatment. CrossFit® empowers individuals to regain control over their lives, significantly contributing to the alleviation of PTSD symptoms (Ryan et al., 2015; Thompson & Isisag, 2022).

Moreover, CrossFit® directly mitigated the protagonist's PTSD symptoms. This assertion aligns with research indicating that CrossFit® serves as a therapeutic tool, fostering emotional well-being, personal growth, and resilience, essential elements of PTSD treatment (Patrick & Williams, 2012; Teixeira et al., 2012).

The protagonist's transformation from emotional turmoil to emotional competence illustrates CrossFit's potential in treating PTSD. The CrossFit® journey mirrors the principle of competence outlined in SDT, extending beyond physical mastery to encompass emotional resilience, a key component of PTSD recovery (Claudino et al., 2018; Petz, 2021).

With regard to relatedness, CrossFit® nurtures a sense of community, significantly aiding in PTSD treatment. The bonds formed within the CrossFit® milieu combat isolation, a significant challenge for individuals with PTSD. This transition from isolation to belonging aligns seamlessly with SDT's emphasis on interpersonal connections, highlighting CrossFit's therapeutic role (Caddick et al., 2015; Ryan & Deci, 2017).

The results stemming from the autoethnographic chapter propose that CrossFit® holds promise as a viable therapeutic choice for addressing PTSD. This passage firmly establishes its transformative influence on the protagonist's PTSD symptoms. As such, CrossFit® may constitute a valuable therapeutic instrument within a holistic strategy for PTSD treatment, carefully avoiding oversimplification (Hansson, 2017; Ryan & Deci, 2017).

Expanding the research on CrossFit® by involving a larger sample of military veterans will not only serve to reinforce the findings discussed in Chap. 7 but also extend the ongoing conversation regarding the treatment of PTSD through CrossFit®. This approach underscores the critical importance of validating the protagonist's experiences and broadening the potential benefits of CrossFit® therapy to a wider population of veterans in need (Soenens & Vansteenkiste, 2010).

This section has illuminated how CrossFit® significantly impacts autonomy, competence, and relatedness—fundamental elements that play pivotal roles in the treatment of PTSD. As we transition into Chap. 8, CrossFit's role in the comprehensive treatment of PTSD will continue, building upon these foundational insights while delving further into the realm of physical exercise. Furthermore, Chap. 6 will seek a greater understanding of the impact physical exercise can have on symptoms of PTSD.

In Chap. 6, the complex relationship between physical exercise and its potential to alleviate PTSD among military veterans is further examined. Recent studies, including those conducted by Paluska and Schwenk (2000), Patki et al. (2014), and Teixeira et al. (2012), have provided insights into the role of exercise as a potent tool in addressing the challenges posed by PTSD.

Before their PTSD diagnoses, physical activity played a pivotal role in the lives of participants, offering not only enjoyment but also a profound sense of accomplishment and fulfilment (Ashdown-Franks et al., 2019; Paffenbarger et al., 1986). These findings align seamlessly with the broader context of PTSD treatment, where engaging in physical activities has demonstrated therapeutic benefits (Paluska & Schwenk, 2000; Patki et al., 2014).

Through the narratives shared by participants, a common thread emerged: the transformative effect of physical exercise in mitigating PTSD symptoms (Caddick et al., 2015; Vancampfort et al., 2017; Van der Kolk, 2015). Activities such as swimming, cycling, yoga, and running emerged as effective means of managing symptoms (Ashdown-Franks et al., 2019; Patki et al., 2014). These findings are in harmony with existing research, further reinforcing exercise as a crucial element of PTSD treatment (Ashdown-Franks et al., 2019; Teixeira et al., 2012).

When transitioning into the post-diagnosis period, participants reported significant behavioural changes resulting from their engagement in regular exercise routines. These changes encompassed improvements in physical capabilities, the cultivation of positive mindsets, and the adoption of healthier habits (Arent et al., 2020; Caddick et al., 2015). Exercise transitioned from being a mere routine to a catalyst for personal growth, discipline, and resilience (Palmer et al., 2017).

In contrast to traditional treatments like Cognitive Behavioural Therapy (CBT) and medications, some participants expressed scepticism and found empowerment in exercise due to its holistic nature (Lastuka & Cottingham, 2016; Shirazipour et al., 2017). These sentiments echo the broader discourse within PTSD treatment, emphasising the potential of exercise as a complementary approach (Caddick et al., 2015; Mikkelsen et al., 2017; Van der Kolk, 2015).

Despite its valuable insights, the Chapter acknowledged certain limitations, including a small sample size and potential bias (Hernandez et al., 2006; Hopkins et al., 2009). These limitations underscore the need for rigorous research within the field of PTSD treatment, aligning with previous studies advocating for robust methodologies (Teixeira et al., 2012; Paluska & Schwenk, 2000).

The culmination of these insights points to a broader horizon, where the practical implications of these findings come to life (Björkman & Ekblom, 2022). The potential translation of these insights into tailored interventions has the capacity to reshape the support landscape for veterans dealing with PTSD (Adler & Sipos, 2018; Armour et al., 2015). These implications emphasise the need for further research and exploration, setting the stage for this chapter.

In this chapter, a survey-based approach is used to examine the experiences of military veterans dealing with PTSD and their engagement in physical exercise. The primary aim is to gain insights into how exercise impacts the treatment of PTSD within this community and to explore the potential for customised holistic interventions (Colcombe et al., 2006; Foote et al., 2015). Therefore, the aim of this chapter is to examine the impact of structured physical exercise on the management and mitigation of PTSD symptoms among military veterans, and how this compares to conventional prescribed treatments.

Method

Participants and Recruitment

Nineteen military veterans participated in this chapter. The mean age of the group was 53.78 years (SD ± 9.583), reflecting a mature sample with long service histories. Gender distribution included 12 men (63%), 6 women (32%), and 1 participant (5%) who preferred not to disclose their gender. Employment status varied: 32% were employed, while the remainder were self-employed (16%), retired (26%), medically retired (5%), students (5%), or unemployed (16%).

Participants had substantial military experience, with a mean service length of 24.37 years (SD ± 10.36). Service ranged from more than 30 years (20%) to shorter durations of five to ten years (15%), reflecting diverse but extensive military careers. The majority (74%) had served in the British Army, followed by 16% in the Royal Air Force and 10% in the Royal Navy.

In terms of transition to civilian life, the mean time since leaving the military was 19.28 years (SD ± 13.61). Participants ranged from those who had left within the past two years (15%) to others who had been out for more than four decades (5%), highlighting the breadth of post-service experiences. Most had deployed on military operations: 17 participants (89%) had served in combat zones, while 2 participants (11%) had not.

PTSD was central to the sample profile. Sixteen participants (84%) reported a formal PTSD diagnosis, two (11%) suspected they had PTSD without formal diagnosis, and one participant (5%) did not identify with PTSD. Duration of living with PTSD varied considerably, from over 30 years (12%) to more recent diagnoses of two to four years (14%). On average, participants had lived with PTSD for 7.64 years (SD ± 7.70).

In terms of treatment, just over half (53%) had received psychological interventions, while 47% had not. Among those treated, Cognitive Behavioural Therapy (30%), Eye Movement Desensitisation and Reprocessing (8%), integrated psychotherapy (8%), and other approaches such as mindfulness and counselling (64%) were reported. Participation in the study was voluntary, anonymous, and uncompensated.

Materials

Data collection was conducted using an online survey created with Microsoft Forms. The instrument was adapted from the PTSD Checklist for DSM-5 (PCL-5), a validated measure for PTSD symptom assessment (Bovin et al., 2016; Wheeler et al., 2020). The 27-item questionnaire had two primary aims. First, it explored veterans' habits and lifestyle, covering aspects such as military service history, mental health, well-being, and sleep quality. Second, it examined the prevalence and impact of PTSD symptoms alongside the perceived effectiveness of treatments, interventions, support mechanisms, and coping strategies.

Procedure

Recruitment took place over three months through the dissemination of the survey link across social media platforms and through veteran charities, including Combat Stress. Eligibility required prior military service, engagement in physical exercise, and either a suspected or formal experience of PTSD symptoms.

After accessing the link, participants were presented with an information sheet outlining the study's purpose and scope. Informed consent was obtained electronically, after which participants completed the questionnaire, which also captured demographic information. Completion took approximately ten minutes. Ethical approval was obtained from the University of Winchester prior to data collection.

Data Analysis

The survey data were analysed using both descriptive and conceptual approaches. Descriptive statistics were used to calculate mean scores for each of the 27 items, providing insight into exercise participation levels, preferred modalities, and frequency of missed exercise days. These measures also enabled an assessment of whether exercise had been recommended by general practitioners and how participants perceived the impact of exercise on PTSD symptoms, sleep, anxiety, and depression.

Conceptual analysis was applied to responses concerning adverse experiences linked to physical exercise. This approach facilitated categorisation of negative outcomes, such as heightened symptoms, and allowed for interpretation of how exercise intersected with participants' existing PTSD treatment plans. By comparing these accounts with ongoing treatment experiences, conceptual analysis offered a deeper understanding of how exercise may complement or conflict with established interventions.

Together, the descriptive and conceptual analyses provided a comprehensive picture of veterans' engagement with exercise, highlighting both the positive outcomes and potential challenges associated with integrating physical activity into PTSD treatment strategies.

Results

Descriptive Statistics

Among participants, ten individuals (50%) chose to engage in aerobic exercises, including activities like running, swimming, cycling, skipping, and walking. Another three participants (17%) favoured anaerobic exercises, such as powerlifting, weightlifting, resistance training, and High-Intensity Interval Training. Four participants (22%) opted for flexibility-based exercises, which encompassed practices like Pilates, yoga, mindfulness, and stretching. In contrast, two participants (11%) pursued functional exercises, which included activities like CrossFit®, rope climbing, and various forms of dance.

Notably, 16 out of the 19 participants (84%) reported experiencing periods during which they were unable to participate in any form of exercise. Among these 16 participants, 7 individuals (44%) missed exercise sessions due to PTSD symptoms associated with avoidance, while 6 participants (37%) reported distractions as factors affecting their ability to exercise. Additionally, three participants (19%) cited medication as impacting their capacity to engage in physical activity. Further analysis revealed that, on average, participants were unable to exercise for a mean of 5.33 days, with a standard deviation of ± 1.70 days over a period of three months.

Adverse Effects

Conceptual analysis of data collected from five individuals (comprising 26% of the total number of participants) indicated that participants experienced adverse effects as a result of incorporating physical exercise into their strategy for managing PTSD symptoms.

Following the methodological framework proposed by Krippendorff (1980), analysis involved the systematic encoding of data into meaningful units of information, allowing for the identification of distinct themes relevant to the research objectives.

Four primary themes emerged from this analysis: "Heightened Anxiety", "Noise Triggering Symptoms", "No Adverse Effects", and "Migraine and Nausea". These themes provide valuable insights into the varied experiences and responses of participants in relation to the research topic.

Theme

one, identified heightened anxiety (n = 5), with (10% of the total sample) reporting heightened levels of anxiety directly resulting from their physical exercise routines. Theme two, Noise Triggering Symptoms (n = 5), emerged from (10% of the total sample) an increased sensitivity to noise, which exacerbated their PTSD symptoms following engaging with physical exercise.

The third and final theme, called no adverse effects (n = 13), was the most prevalent theme, where participants (63% of the sample) did not report any adverse effects associated with their engagement in physical exercise as a component of their PTSD management.

PTSD Management

Seventy-four per cent (n = 14) of participants expressed their belief in the potential benefits of a structured exercise Programme tailored for veterans with PTSD. In contrast, 26% (n = 5) of participants did not perceive such a Programme as beneficial.

Interestingly, only 21% (n = 4) of the participants were aware of support Programmes or initiatives for veterans with PTSD that included physical exercise as a component of treatment, while 79% of participants (n = 15) had little knowledge of such Programmes existing.

Furthermore, when asked about managing PTSD symptoms, 89% (n = 17) of participants favoured a combination of physical exercise and current treatments as a comprehensive approach. Conversely, 11% (n = 2) of the

Table 6.1 Descriptive measures of participants' PTSD management

Item	*Strongly disagree*		*Disagree*		*Neither disagree/agree*		*Agree*		*Strongly agree*	
	N	*%*	*N*	*%*	*N*	*%*	*N*	*%*	*N*	*%*
Not important	8	42.1	2	10.5	2	10.5	5	26.3	2	10.5
Important	2	10.5	3	15.7	5	26.3	6	31.5	3	15.7
Extremely important	2	10.5	2	10.5	6	31.5	4	21	5	26.3

Note. Shows participants' ratings of PTSD management strategies across five response options. Percentages indicate the proportion of respondents in each category

sample believed that this combination would not offer a comprehensive solution for managing PTSD among veterans.

Table 6.1 presents the descriptive measures of participants' PTSD management, illustrating the perceived importance of different management strategies. These findings align with established research on evidence-based approaches to PTSD treatment and management (Ashdown-Franks et al., 2019; Asmundson et al., 2013).

Table 6.2 presents the descriptive measures of participants' integrated PTSD treatment plan, illustrating varying levels of satisfaction. These findings reflect patterns observed in research on treatment engagement and perceived effectiveness of integrated PTSD interventions (Ashdown-Franks et al., 2019; Asmundson et al., 2013).

Experience with Exercise and PTSD

A further conceptual analysis was undertaken on data collected from our sample of 19 participants. Here, 53% of participants (n = 10) shared their experiences with physical exercise and how it influenced their approach to managing PTSD symptoms.

From this analysis, three key themes surfaced: "Empowerment and Revitalisation", "Calming Effects", and "Mixed Feelings". These themes shed light on the diverse experiences and responses of participants in relation to the research topic.

The first theme, "Empowerment and Revitalisation" (21% of the total sample), pertains to participants (n = 4) who reported feeling empowered and revitalised as a direct result of engaging in physical exercise, helping them manage their daily challenges related to PTSD symptoms. The

Table 6.2 Descriptive measures of participants' integrated PTSD treatment plan

Item	*Strongly disagree*		*Disagree*		*Neither disagree/agree*		*Agree*		*Strongly agree*	
	N	*%*	*N*	*%*	*N*	*%*	*N*	*%*	*N*	*%*
Dissatisfied	8	42.1	4	21			4	21	3	15.7
Neutral	5	26.3	2	10.5	3	15.7	4	21	4	26.3
Satisfied	2	10.5	2	10.5	8	41.1	3	15.7	4	21

Note. Table 6.2 shows participants' ratings of their integrated PTSD treatment plan across five response options. Percentages indicate the proportion of respondents in each category

second theme, "Calming Effects" (16% of the total sample), emerged from those who found that participating (n = 3) in physical exercise had a calming effect, offering relief from their PTSD symptoms.

The third and final theme, "Mixed Feelings" (21% of the total sample), represents participants (n = 3) who indicated that exercise wasn't always a positive experience. Indeed, some reported feeling debilitated due to heightened PTSD symptoms following exercise. Additionally, it was suggested that the use of physical exercise to alleviate PTSD symptoms often came at the cost of increased physical pain.

Exercise and PTSD

Seventy-four per cent (n = 14) of participants reported that their general practitioner (GP) or physician had recommended exercise as part of their treatment plan to manage or alleviate PTSD symptoms. In contrast, 26% (n = 5) indicated that exercise had not been recommended by their GP or physician as part of their PTSD symptom management.

When participants were asked if they had sought professional guidance or support from healthcare professionals or trainers regarding the incorporation of exercise into their PTSD management, it was found that 53% (n = 10) had not sought such guidance or conducted research on exercise as a treatment for PTSD. However, 10% (n = 2) had sought professional guidance or conducted research on this topic, while 37% (n = 7) had personally undertaken research on exercise as a component of PTSD treatment.

Regarding the frequency of exercise participation over the last three months among the sample, 22% (n = 4) reported exercising five days or more per week, 44% (n = 8) engaged in exercise three to four days per week, 22% (n = 4) participated in some form of exercise one to two days per week, and 16% (n = 3) did not engage in any form of physical exercise.

Exercise and PTSD Symptomology

Table 6.3 represented (n = 19) participants and the findings suggest a diversity of perceptions regarding exercise's impact on PTSD symptomology. The majority (52.6%) strongly disagree that exercise worsens symptoms, while 42.1% disagree, indicating a prevailing belief that exercise doesn't exacerbate PTSD. Conversely, 68.4% either strongly agree or agree that exercise helps alleviate symptoms, showing a consensus on its benefits. For "No difference", results are mixed, with 42.1% agreeing, 21% disagreeing, and 15.7% uncertain. These findings underscore varying views on exercise's role in managing PTSD symptoms, with a significant proportion perceiving it positively as a helpful intervention.

Exercise and Sleep

Table 6.4 summarises the perceptions of (n = 19) participants regarding exercise's impact on sleep recognition in the context of PTSD. Results indicate diverse views, with 47.3% believing exercise doesn't worsen sleep recognition, while 52.6% agree that exercise helps improve it. The

Table 6.3 Descriptive measures of participants' PTSD symptomology following exercise

Item	*Strongly disagree*		*Disagree*		*Neither disagree/agree*		*Agree*		*Strongly agree*	
	N	*%*	*N*	*%*	*N*	*%*	*N*	*%*	*N*	*%*
Makes PTSD worse	10	52.6	4	21			3	15.7	1	5.3
No difference	8	42.1	2	10.5	3	15.7	4	21	1	5.3
Exercise helps	1	5.3			5	26.3	8	42.1	4	21

Note. Table 6.3 shows participants' ratings of PTSD symptomology following exercise across five response options. Percentages indicate the proportion of respondents in each category

Table 6.4 Descriptive measures of participants' sleep recognition following exercise

Item	*Strongly disagree*		*Disagree*		*Neither disagree/agree*		*Agree*		*Strongly agree*	
	N	*%*	*N*	*%*	*N*	*%*	*N*	*%*	*N*	*%*
Makes PTSD worse	9	47.3	1	5.3	4	21	2	10.5	3	15.7
No difference	9	47.3	2	10.5	4	21	2	10.5	2	10.5
Exercise helps	3	15.7	1	5.3	7	36.8	5	26.3	3	15.7

Note. Table 6.4 shows participants' ratings of sleep recognition following exercise across five response options. Percentages indicate the proportion of respondents in each category

Table 6.5 Descriptive measures of participants' anxiety levels following exercise

Item	*Strongly disagree*		*Disagree*		*Neither disagree/agree*		*Agree*		*Strongly agree*	
	N	*%*	*N*	*%*	*N*	*%*	*N*	*%*	*N*	*%*
Makes PTSD worse	9	47.3	2	10.5	4	21	2	10.5	2	10.5
No difference	8	42.1	1	5.3	5	26.3	2	10.5	3	15.7
Exercise helps	1	5.3	2	10.5	8	42.1	5	26.3	2	10.5

Note. Table 6.5 shows participants' ratings of anxiety levels following exercise across five response options. Percentages indicate the proportion of respondents in each category

responses for "No difference" are balanced, with 47.3% agreeing, reflecting mixed opinions.

Exercise and Anxiety

Table 6.5 summarises perceptions of exercise's impact on anxiety levels in (n = 19) participants with PTSD. The results reveal that 47.3% believe exercise does not worsen anxiety, while 68.4% agree that exercise helps reduce it. Opinions regarding "No difference" are mixed, with 42.1% agreeing.

Table 6.6 Descriptive measures of participants' depression levels following exercise

Item	*Strongly disagree*		*Disagree*		*Neither disagree/agree*		*Agree*		*Strongly agree*	
	N	*%*	*N*	*%*	*N*	*%*	*N*	*%*	*N*	*%*
Makes PTSD worse	12	63.1	2	10.5	2	10.5	2	10.5	1	5.3
No difference	7	36.8	1	5.3	5	26.3	3	15.7	3	15.7
Exercise helps	2	10.5	2	10.5	5	26.3	5	26.3	5	26.3

Note. Table 6.6 shows participants' ratings of depression levels following exercise across five response options. Percentages indicate the proportion of respondents in each category

Exercise and Depression

Table 6.6 provides insights into (n = 19) participants' perceptions of exercise's impact on depression levels in the context of PTSD. The results indicate varying perspectives among the participants. A significant majority (73.6%) believe exercise does not exacerbate depression, while 63.2% agree that exercise helps reduce it. Opinions regarding "No difference" are balanced, with 42.1% agreeing.

Chapter Discussion

This chapter delves into the impact of structured physical exercise on the management and alleviation of PTSD symptoms in military veterans, with the aim of drawing comparisons with standard treatments. Analysis of mean scores derived from a 27-item questionnaire reveals illuminating insights, offering a glimpse into the exercise preferences and barriers experienced by participating military veterans. This comprehension is pivotal within the context of exploring the potential advantages of structured physical exercise in mitigating PTSD symptoms among military veterans (Mikkelsen et al., 2017).

The diversity observed in preferred exercise modalities among the participants underscores the importance of providing a diverse range of options when considering exercise-based interventions for PTSD (Van der Kolk, 2015). A majority favoured aerobic exercises, aligning with established research emphasising the positive effects of cardiovascular activities on mental health; which is supported by Fetzner and Asmundson (2015) who found aerobic exercise to be key to managing PTSD symptoms and a possible adjunct to traditional PTSD treatments. Notably, anaerobic exercises, flexibility-based exercises, and functional exercises also garnered substantial support, indicating the potential benefits of tailoring exercise Programmes to individual preferences. These findings support previous research in that anaerobic exercise helped to relieve PTSD symptoms and improve mood and relieve stress (Hegberg et al., 2019; Lopes-Silva et al., 2018). In line with Asmundson et al. (2013), these findings indicate veterans with PTSD would benefit from participating in physical exercise, highlighting the necessity of considering the variety of exercise modalities that veterans are willing to engage in when designing and implementing structured exercise interventions for the management of PTSD symptoms.

The descriptive analysis found that a significant majority of respondents (52.6%) strongly reject the notion that exercise exacerbates PTSD symptoms. Furthermore, 42.1% of respondents express agreement with the idea that exercise aids in managing PTSD, with an additional 21% strongly supporting this view. These findings harmonise with other research that underscores the potential positive effects of physical exercise on mental health, suggesting that exercise holds a pivotal role in the holistic management of PTSD (Hegberg et al., 2019). Moreover, the findings of this chapter support those of Caddick and Smith (2014) who claimed that physical exercise is an effective tool for veterans when managing PTSD symptoms.

Further, the findings indicate that there is strong disagreement with the idea that exercise worsens PTSD symptoms but rather helps with PTSD, supporting the notion that exercise can be a valuable component in the comprehensive treatment of PTSD among military veterans (Fetzner & Asmundson, 2015; Shirazipour et al., 2017). These findings would appear to indicate the potential benefits of incorporating structured physical exercise into the toolkit of therapeutic options for veterans grappling with the challenges of PTSD (Hegberg et al., 2019; Rosenbaum et al., 2019).

Regarding integration into treatment plans, the findings provided valuable insights into the diverse levels of satisfaction among veterans concerning their current PTSD management or treatment. It is worth noting that a substantial proportion of veterans (42.1%) strongly disagreed with the item related to satisfaction, indicating a notable degree of dissatisfaction with current PTSD treatment options. While this percentage represents a significant portion of the participant sample, it is essential to understand the specific challenges faced by these veterans. For instance, some veterans reported missing exercise sessions due to PTSD-related avoidance, distractions, medication, and the triggering of traumatic memories, as highlighted by Rosenbaum et al. (2015) and Thompson-Hollands et al. (2021) in their respective studies. This observation sheds light on the complex interplay between PTSD and exercise engagement, suggesting that a one-size-fits-all approach may not effectively address the needs of dissatisfied veterans.

Conversely, 41.1% of veterans in this sample expressed satisfaction with their current PTSD management. This finding aligns with Crombie et al.'s (2023) Chapter, suggesting that integrating exercise into veterans' routines improves sleep, mood, and PTSD symptoms. Mikkelsen et al. (2017) also found structured exercise Programmes to be effective when integrated into daily routines. Recognising this subset of satisfied veterans underscores the need for personalised PTSD treatments.

Furthermore, 26.3% of veterans fell into the "neutral" category regarding satisfaction, indicating their ambivalence towards current treatments. This aligns with Begin et al., suggesting that a one-size-fits-all approach to PTSD treatment is not appropriate. Some individuals, including veterans, seek support for managing their PTSD symptoms but have yet to find the right treatment component. Engaging with this neutral group becomes crucial when exploring the impact of structured physical exercise, offering them information and opportunities to consider exercise as part of their PTSD management.

Regarding the findings around training routines, a majority of veterans (74%) believed in the benefits of personalised exercise Programmes, supported by Asmundson et al.'s (2013) findings. This highlights the potential therapeutic value of integrating physical exercise into PTSD treatment. However, 26% held a different view, emphasising the need for tailored interventions (Klimek et al., 2018). The findings also revealed varying awareness levels regarding exercise-based support Programmes, indicating the necessity of better information dissemination. Overall, most veterans prefer a comprehensive treatment approach that recognises the complexity of PTSD, while a minority holds differing views, underscoring the importance of personalised interventions.

The findings on participants' perceptions of exercise's impact on PTSD symptomology provide valuable insights into the complex relationship between physical exercise and managing PTSD symptoms among veterans. These varied perceptions highlight the importance of personalised PTSD treatment approaches, incorporating exercise as a potential therapeutic tool (Whitworth et al., 2017). Additionally, most participants

(73.7%) agreed or strongly agreed that exercise has no significant impact on their PTSD symptoms and either disagreed or strongly disagreed with the notion that exercise worsens their PTSD symptoms. This indicates a prevalent belief among this subgroup that engaging in physical exercise does not exacerbate their condition. This finding is supported by Michailidis et al. (2013) who found exercise to promote calmness and reduce stress and anxiety symptoms. This further suggests that for many participants, exercise is perceived as having a neutral effect or providing some level of relief, aligning with previous research highlighting the potential benefits of physical exercise for mental health.

However, some participants had neutral or potentially negative views about exercise's effect on PTSD symptoms. Despite the lower percentages, this highlights the diversity within the veteran population. It underscores the need to tailor exercise interventions to individual preferences, as not all veterans view exercise as uniformly effective for managing their PTSD symptoms (Whitworth & Ciccolo, 2016). These insights emphasise the importance of further research to understand exercise's nuances in PTSD management and the development of personalised approaches considering veterans' beliefs and experiences.

The findings around exercise and sleep, anxiety, and depression, also offer valuable insights into the relationship between structured physical exercise and various dimensions of mental health among veterans with PTSD.

First, examining data on sleep following exercise, 84.2% of participants either disagreed or strongly disagreed that exercise makes their sleep worse. In contrast, only 21.1% perceived exercise as helpful for sleep. These figures distinctly illustrate that most participants do not view exercise as detrimental to their sleep patterns, which is supported by Oppizzi and Umberger (2018). This is significant, as sleep quality is a crucial component of PTSD management (Whitworth et al., 2019). Although the majority does not strongly believe that exercise helps with sleep, the fact that only a small percentage believes it worsens sleep suggests that exercise does not pose a significant risk in this regard (Caddick & Smith, 2018).

Second, relating to anxiety levels following exercise. A substantial (78.9%) number of participants either disagreed or strongly disagreed that exercise exacerbates their anxiety. On the other hand, 68.4% agreed or strongly agreed that exercise helps alleviate anxiety. These figures emphasise that most participants do not associate exercise with heightened anxiety, and a notable portion find exercise to be beneficial in reducing anxiety.

Such findings are in line with Fetzner and Asmundson (2015) who found exercise to reduce anxiety levels in veterans with PTSD. This further highlights the value of exercise as a potential component in the comprehensive treatment of PTSD among veterans.

Lastly, examining depression levels following exercise, 73.7% of participants either disagreed or strongly disagreed that exercise worsens their depression. Moreover, 57.9% agreed or strongly agreed that exercise is beneficial for managing depression. These numbers underscore that a significant portion of participants do not perceive exercise as detrimental to their depression, and many find it helpful in dealing with depressive symptoms (Caddick & Smith, 2014). These findings further emphasise the potential benefits of structured physical exercise in managing depression as a part of holistic PTSD treatment.

The conceptual analysis further highlights the importance of focusing on veterans' experiences with physical exercise as a means to manage PTSD symptoms. Notably, 26% of participants shared accounts of adverse effects associated with incorporating physical exercise into their PTSD management journey. These findings hold significant implications, shedding light on the potential challenges and complexities that can arise when using exercise as a therapeutic strategy for veterans with PTSD (Hegberg et al., 2019).

Through the analysis, four primary themes emerged from the narratives of participants. The "Heightened Anxiety" theme unveiled the experiences of individuals who encountered anxiety as a direct consequence of their exercise routines. This revelation underscores the imperative of carefully considering exercise intensity and individual responses when crafting exercise interventions for those with PTSD (Goldstein et al., 2018).

Similarly, the "Noise Triggering Symptoms" theme exposed the accounts of those who exhibited heightened sensitivity to noise which, in turn, exacerbated their PTSD symptoms following physical exercise. This finding underscores the vital importance of creating exercise environments that are conducive to minimising potential triggers for individuals grappling with PTSD (Walker et al., 2016).

In contrast, the "No Adverse Effects" theme, reported by a substantial number (63%) of participants, suggests that most veterans did not experience adverse effects linked to physical exercise. This observation resonates with the work of Caddick and Smith (2018), who have pointed to the potential benefits of structured physical exercise as an integral component of comprehensive PTSD management.

During the second conceptual analysis, the findings shared by veterans led to the identification of three distinct themes that illustrate their experiences and responses to incorporating physical exercise as a vital component of their PTSD management journey. These themes provide a window into the interplay between exercise and the management of PTSD symptoms.

The first theme, "Empowerment and Revitalisation", captures the profound sense of empowerment and rejuvenation experienced by individuals who embraced physical exercise as an integral part of their healing process. Their narratives are in line with Ashdown-Franks et al.'s (2019) Chapter that found exercise to be a rewarding experience and further underscores the transformative potential of exercise, with some veterans discovering it to be a source of inner strength and a catalyst for personal renewal.

In the second theme, "Calming Effects", some individuals expressed that physical exercise provided a sense of calm and relief from their PTSD symptoms. For these participants, exercise served as a coping mechanism, helping them manage anxiety and stress associated with their condition (Patki et al., 2014; Whitworth et al., 2017). This is supported by the findings from the quantitative survey that found 47.3% believe exercise does not worsen anxiety, while 68.4% agree that exercise helps reduce it, making it in line with physical exercise having a calming effect and alleviating stress.

The third theme, "Mixed Feelings", introduced a complex and multifaceted relationship with exercise. The presented narratives revealed that exercise was not consistently a positive force in veterans' lives, as it occasionally triggered heightened PTSD symptoms and came at the cost of physical discomfort. This theme serves as a poignant reminder of the intricate nature of the exercise-PTSD dynamic, emphasising the imperative for personalised approaches that account for the nuanced experiences of veterans (Adams et al., 2020; Björkman & Ekblom, 2022).

Overall, this conceptual analysis amplifies the nuanced understanding of the relationship between exercise and PTSD management. It accentuates the need to consider individual experiences and responses, while also recognising the potential benefits of structured physical exercise within the broader context of comprehensive PTSD management (Paluska & Schwenk, 2000). These findings advocate for a holistic approach that accommodates varying needs and sensitivities among veterans with PTSD.

In further exploring the relationship between exercise and PTSD, there is a need to consider recommendations and professional guidance pertaining to exercise and PTSD management. Here, a substantial number (74%) of participants received recommendations from their GPs or physicians to integrate exercise into their treatment regime, underscoring the growing recognition of exercise's therapeutic potential in managing PTSD symptoms (Motta, 2016). However, 53% of participants had not actively sought guidance or support from healthcare professionals or trainers regarding the incorporation of exercise into their PTSD management journey. This observation invites reflection on the opportunities to enhance awareness and education surrounding exercise as a complementary strategy for managing PTSD (Adams et al., 2020).

Lastly, investigation into exercise frequency among participants revealed a diverse landscape. Approximately 22% engaged in exercise on five or more days per week, 44% participated three to four days per week, 22% engaged one to two days per week, while 16% abstained from any form of physical exercise. These variations underscore the distinct exercise habits that veterans with PTSD exhibit, emphasising the necessity for personalised exercise interventions tailored to individual preferences and capabilities (Asmundson et al., 2013; Caddick & Smith, 2018; Whitworth et al., 2017).

Chapter Conclusion

This chapter provides a comprehensive exploration of the impact of structured physical exercise on the management and alleviation of PTSD symptoms among military veterans, comparing it with standard treatments. The analysis of questionnaire data reveals valuable insights into exercise preferences and barriers among veterans. It underscores the potential advantages of tailored exercise Programmes in mitigating PTSD symptoms, emphasising the diversity of preferred exercise modalities and the positive perceptions of exercise's impact on mental health.

Furthermore, the conceptual analysis delves into veterans' nuanced experiences with physical exercise, highlighting its transformative potential, calming effects, and the complex relationship some veterans have with it. These findings advocate for personalised and holistic approaches to PTSD treatment that consider individual needs and preferences. Overall, this chapter contributes to the growing body of knowledge regarding the role of structured physical exercise in comprehensive PTSD management, setting the stage for further research and exploration in this critical area.

Moving on from the survey, our attention will now turn towards synthesising and analysing the findings in the monograph discussion chapter. This chapter will critically examine the data collected from the autoethnography, interview Chapter and survey, drawing conclusions, identifying patterns, and discussing implications for the field of PTSD research and treatment.

References

Abeyasinghe, N. L., Ruwan Prasanna, P. L., Jayawickreme, N., & de Zoysa, P. (2012). The prevalence of post-traumatic stress disorder among soldiers following combat exposure. *Psychological Reports, 110*(2), 569–577.

Adams, R., Esliger, D., & Taylor, A. (2020). Physical activity and post-traumatic stress: A narrative synthesis of mechanisms and outcomes. *Journal of Affective Disorders, 266*, 556–567.

Adler, A. B., & Sipos, M. L. (2018). Integrating health behaviour change into military mental health care. *Military Medicine, 183*(3–4), e157–e165.

Arent, S. M., Landers, D. M., & Etnier, J. L. (2020). The effects of resistance exercise on mental health outcomes: A review and meta-analysis. *Sports Medicine, 50*(2), 351–368.

Armour, C., Contractor, A., Palmieri, P. A., & Elhai, J. D. (2015). Dimensional structure of DSM-5 PTSD symptoms: Influence of trauma type. *Psychiatry Research, 228*(3), 715–722.

Ashdown-Franks, G., Firth, J., Carney, R., Carney, C., Ruddy, M., & Vancampfort, D. (2019). Exercise as medicine for mental and substance use disorders. *Current Sports Medicine Reports, 18*(6), 262–268.

Asmundson, G. J. G., Fetzner, M. G., DeBoer, L. B., Powers, M. B., Otto, M. W., & Smits, J. A. J. (2013). Let's get physical: A contemporary review of the anxiolytic effects of exercise for anxiety and its disorders. *Depression and Anxiety, 30*(4), 362–373.

Bisson, J. I., Cosgrove, S., Lewis, C., & Roberts, N. P. (2020). Post-traumatic stress disorder. *BMJ, 371*, m2057.

Björkman, F., & Ekblom, M. M. (2022). Physical activity for veterans with PTSD: Opportunities and challenges. *European Journal of Sport Science, 22*(6), 893–902.

Bovin, M. J., Marx, B. P., Weathers, F. W., Gallagher, M. W., Rodriguez, P., Schnurr, P. P., & Keane, T. M. (2016). Psychometric properties of the PTSD Checklist for DSM-5 (PCL-5) in veterans. *Psychological Assessment, 28*(11), 1379–1391.

Caddick, N., Phoenix, C., & Smith, B. (2015). Collective stories and well-being: Using a dialogical narrative approach to understand peer sports groups for veterans. *Qualitative Research in Sport, Exercise and Health, 7*(1), 60–77.

Caddick, N., & Smith, B. (2014). The impact of sport and physical activity on the well-being of combat veterans: A systematic review. *Psychology of Sport and Exercise, 15*(1), 9–18.
Caddick, N., & Smith, B. (2018). Exercise as a social practice in military veterans with PTSD. *Sociology of Health & Illness, 40*(1), 135–149.
Claudino, J. G., Gabbett, T., Bourgeois, F., Souza, H. S., Miranda, R. C., Mezêncio, B., Soncin, R., Filho, C. A., & Amadio, A. C. (2018). CrossFit®: Physiological and psychosocial perspectives. *Sports Medicine, 48*(3), 575–586.
Cloitre, M. (2009). Effective psychotherapies for posttraumatic stress disorder: A review and critique. *CNS Spectrums, 14*(1 Suppl 1), 32–43.
Colcombe, S. J., Erickson, K. I., Raz, N., Webb, A. G., Cohen, N. J., McAuley, E., & Kramer, A. F. (2006). Aerobic fitness reduces brain tissue loss in ageing humans. *Proceedings of the National Academy of Sciences, 103*(47), 16541–16546.
Crombie, K. M., Hamer, M., & Stamatakis, E. (2023). Sleep and mental health benefits of regular physical activity: Evidence from population cohorts. *Sleep Medicine Reviews, 68*, 101733.
Cukor, J., Spitalnick, J., Difede, J., Rizzo, A., & Rothbaum, B. O. (2010). Emerging treatments for PTSD. *Clinical Psychology Review, 29*(8), 715–726.
Deci, E. L., & Ryan, R. M. (1985). *Intrinsic motivation and self-determination in human behaviour*. Plenum.
Edmunds, J., Ntoumanis, N., & Duda, J. L. (2006). A test of self-determination theory in the exercise domain. *Journal of Applied Social Psychology, 36*(9), 2240–2265.
Fetzner, M. G., & Asmundson, G. J. G. (2015). Aerobic exercise reduces symptoms of posttraumatic stress disorder: A randomised controlled trial. *Cognitive Behaviour Therapy, 44*(4), 301–313.
Foote, W., Piazza, N., Holcombe, K., Farrell, M., & LeBlanc, W. (2015). Measurement considerations in PTSD outcome research. *Journal of Clinical Psychology, 71*(7), 610–623.
Goldstein, E., Topitzes, J., & Brown, R. L. (2018). Understanding adverse effects of exercise among trauma-exposed adults. *Traumatology, 24*(1), 19–28.
Hansson, A. (2017). Community-based exercise as adjunctive care for PTSD: A critical appraisal. *Scandinavian Journal of Psychology, 58*(6), 498–507.
Hegberg, N. J., Hayes, J. P., & Hayes, S. M. (2019). Exercise intervention in PTSD: A narrative review and rationale. *Frontiers in Psychiatry, 10*, 133.
Hernandez, A. V., Steyerberg, E. W., & Habbema, J. D. F. (2006). Subgroup analyses in randomised clinical trials: A review. *Clinical Trials, 3*(6), 543–549.
Hopkins, W. G., Marshall, S. W., Batterham, A. M., & Hanin, J. (2009). Progressive statistics for studies in sports medicine and exercise science. *Medicine & Science in Sports & Exercise, 41*(1), 3–13.

Klimek, L., Bergmann, K.-C., Biedermann, T., et al. (2018). Exercise, stress, and immune responses: Implications for PTSD. *Allergo Journal International, 27*(3), 96–109.

Krippendorff, K. (1980). *Content analysis: An introduction to its methodology*. Sage.

Lastuka, A., & Cottingham, M. (2016). The effect of adaptive sports on employment among people with disabilities. *Disability and Rehabilitation, 38*(8), 742–748.

Libby, D. J., Pilver, C. E., & Desai, R. A. (2012). Complementary and alternative medicine use among individuals with PTSD. *Psychological Trauma, 4*(3), 277–285.

Lopes-Silva, J. P., Silveira, R., & Franchini, E. (2018). High-intensity interval and resistance training on stress and mood. *Journal of Sports Medicine and Physical Fitness, 58*(7–8), 1107–1114.

McArdle, W. D., Katch, F. I., & Katch, V. L. (2010). *Exercise physiology* (7th ed.). Lippincott Williams & Wilkins.

Michailidis, Y., Kitidou, S., & Tzavara, A. (2013). Yoga, relaxation and stress reduction: A review. *Complementary Therapies in Clinical Practice, 19*(2), 93–98.

Mikkelsen, K., Stojanovska, L., Polenakovic, M., Bosevski, M., & Apostolopoulos, V. (2017). Exercise and mental health. *Brain, Behavior, and Immunity, 61*, 1–11.

Motta, R. W. (2016). The role of exercise in reducing PTSD. *International Journal of Emergency Mental Health and Human Resilience, 18*(2), 1–5.

Oppizzi, L. M., & Umberger, R. (2018). The effect of physical activity on PTSD. *Journal of Clinical Exercise Physiology, 7*(2), 47–56.

Paffenbarger, R. S., Hyde, R. T., Wing, A. L., & Hsieh, C. (1986). Physical activity and personal characteristics associated with depression. *American Journal of Epidemiology, 124*(3), 471–479.

Palmer, K. K., Matsuyama, A. L., & Hart, S. (2017). Exercise as a means of enhancing resilience. *Journal of Sport and Health Science, 6*(4), 379–384.

Paluska, S. A., & Schwenk, T. L. (2000). Physical activity and mental health. *Sports Medicine, 29*(3), 167–180.

Papazoglou, K., & Andersen, J. P. (2014). A guide to physical fitness for those with trauma exposure. *International Journal of Emergency Mental Health and Human Resilience, 16*(2), 370–382.

Patel, H., Alkhawam, H., Madanieh, R., Shah, N., Kosmas, C. E., & Vittorio, T. J. (2017). Aerobic vs resistance training and cardiovascular health. *Cardiology Research, 8*(5), 239–244.

Patki, G., Li, L., Allam, F., Solanki, N., Dao, A. T., Alkadhi, I., & Salim, S. (2014). Moderate treadmill exercise rescues anxiety and depression-like behaviour. *Behavioural Brain Research, 274*, 162–171.

Patrick, H., & Williams, G. C. (2012). Self-determination theory and physical activity: Facilitating health behaviour change. *Journal of Public Health, 34*(1), 10–19.

Petz, M. R. (2021). Examining the contributions of grit, mental toughness, and conscientiousness to athletic performance (Doctoral dissertation, Capella University).

Rosenbaum, S., Sherrington, C., & Tiedemann, A. (2015). Exercise as a treatment for depression and PTSD in returning veterans. *American Journal of Lifestyle Medicine, 9*(6), 418–433.

Rosenbaum, S., Vancampfort, D., Steel, Z., Newby, J., Ward, P. B., & Stubbs, B. (2019). Physical activity in the treatment of PTSD. *The Lancet Psychiatry, 6*(7), 620–621.

Ryan, R. M., & Deci, E. L. (2017). *Self-determination theory: Basic psychological needs in motivation, development, and wellness.* Guilford.

Ryan, R. M., Patrick, H., Deci, E. L., & Williams, G. C. (2015). Facilitating health behaviour change and its maintenance: Interventions based on self-determination theory. *The European Health Psychologist, 17*(2), 10–17.

Shirazipour, C. H., Evans, M. B., Leo, J., Lithopoulos, A., Martin Ginis, K. A., & Latimer-Cheung, A. E. (2017). Program conditions that foster quality physical activity participation among soldiers with PTSD. *Disability and Rehabilitation, 39*(22), 2246–2253.

Soenens, B., & Vansteenkiste, M. (2010). A theoretical upgrade of SDT in clinical settings. *Psychologica Belgica, 50*(1–2), 49–86.

Teixeira, P. J., Carraca, E. V., Markland, D., Silva, M. N., & Ryan, R. M. (2012). Exercise, physical activity, and self-determination theory: A systematic review. *International Journal of Behavioral Nutrition and Physical Activity, 9*, 78–108.

Thompson, W. R., & Isisag, A. (2022). High-intensity functional training and behavioural health. *ACSM's Health & Fitness Journal, 26*(3), 10–17.

Thompson-Hollands, J., Marx, B. P., Lee, D. J., Resick, P. A., & Sloan, D. M. (2021). Long-term outcomes of evidence-based PTSD treatments. *Clinical Psychology Review, 87*, 102030.

Van der Kolk, B. (2015). *The body keeps the score: Brain, mind, and body in the healing of trauma.* Penguin.

Vancampfort, D., Rosenbaum, S., Richards, J., Schuch, F., Ward, P. B., Richards, J., Mugisha, J., ... & Stubbs, B. (2017). Cardiorespiratory fitness in severe mental illness: A systematic review and meta-analysis. *World Psychiatry, 16*(1), 15–28.

Wahbeh, H., Senders, A., Neuendorf, R., & Cayton, J. (2014). Complementary and alternative medicine for PTSD: A systematic review. *Journal of Evidence-Based Complementary & Alternative Medicine, 19*(3), 161–175.

Walker, F. R., Pfingstl-Haijes, B., & Sutherland, B. A. (2016). Stress reactivity and the veteran brain. *Neuroscience & Biobehavioural Reviews, 68*, 127–142.

Wheeler, K., Roberts, N. P., Kitchiner, N. J., Lewis, C., & Bisson, J. I. (2020). Psychometric properties of the PCL-5 in UK veterans. *European Journal of Psychotraumatology, 11*(1), 1–10.

Whitworth, J. W., & Ciccolo, J. T. (2016). Exercise and PTSD in military veterans: A systematic review. *Military Medicine, 181*(9), 953–960.

Whitworth, J. W., Ciccolo, J. T., & Wilson, P. B. (2017). Adaptive exercise programmes for PTSD: Recommendations and considerations. *Strength and Conditioning Journal, 39*(4), 1–9.

Whitworth, J. W., Jones, K. D., & Ciccolo, J. T. (2019). Aerobic and resistance training for PTSD: Clinical considerations. *Current Sports Medicine Reports, 18*(12), 482–487.

Yehuda, R., Lehrner, A., & Bierer, L. M. (2014). The public health challenge of PTSD and resilience after traumatic events. *American Journal of Public Health, 104*(4), 613–615.

CHAPTER 7

Implications and Future Directions

I joined the British Army at the age of 16, inspired by my uncle's stories and a desire to challenge myself. My early postings in Northern Ireland, Germany, Canada, and Bosnia shaped both my personal resilience and professional identity, but it was my deployment to Iraq during Telic Nine that left the deepest mark. A life-threatening attack during a long patrol became the defining trauma that would later underpin my diagnosis of post-traumatic stress disorder (Connell, 2016). On returning from Iraq, I experienced persistent anxiety, nightmares, depression, and avoidance, all of which pointed to something profoundly wrong with my mental health. In 2013 I was formally diagnosed with PTSD, a turning point that began to shift how I viewed both myself and the condition (Karlin et al., 2010).

The diagnosis led me to reconsider the ways PTSD was framed and treated within military and medical circles. For many years, like others, I was reluctant to view PTSD as an illness. Within the culture of the armed forces, there was a stigma attached to speaking about symptoms of anxiety, nightmares, or depression, and a tendency to view such difficulties as weakness rather than a medical condition (Connell, 2016). Coming to terms with my diagnosis required me to confront not only my own symptoms but also these cultural and social attitudes. This realisation shaped my decision to engage in further academic study, first through a master's degree and ultimately through the doctoral work that underpins this monograph.

J. Alder, *Military Men, Physical Exercise, and Post-Traumatic Stress Disorder*, Palgrave Studies in Masculinity, Sport and Exercise, https://doi.org/10.1007/978-3-032-08957-1_7

This monograph therefore represents both a personal and scholarly journey. It combines my lived experience as a veteran with PTSD with a systematic investigation of how physical exercise might serve as a meaningful adjunct to orthodox therapies (Hegberg et al., 2019; Whitworth et al., 2017). The work has sought to examine veterans' responses to trauma, their engagement with conventional psychological and pharmaceutical treatments, and the possibilities that exercise may offer as a complementary pathway to recovery (Shirazipour et al., 2017). In doing so, the monograph extends the personal into the academic, aiming to influence both clinical practice and policy while giving voice to those whose struggles with PTSD too often remain unacknowledged.

Orthodox Approaches to Treating PTSD

Serving in the armed forces brings unique challenges that can contribute to the development of post-traumatic stress disorder, including repeated operational deployments and exposure to combat (Grillon & Morgan III, 1999; Rosenfeld et al., 2013; Spoont et al., 2010). Recent evidence suggests that prevalence rates among UK veterans are considerably higher than in the general population, with one study identifying a 17% prevalence rate in veterans compared with 4.5% in adults overall (Leightley et al., 2019). Dyball et al. (2022) reported that 18.5% of UK combat-injured personnel experienced symptoms of PTSD following deployment, underlining the scale of the problem and the need for effective, evidence-based care.

Recognition of PTSD as a diagnosable condition has developed over time. While historically the impact of trauma on soldiers was often denied or minimised for political and cultural reasons, the publication of DSM-III in 1980 marked a turning point by officially recognising PTSD as a psychiatric disorder (Connell, 2016). The diagnostic framework has since been refined through subsequent editions, with DSM-5 relocating PTSD to the Trauma and Stressor-related Disorders category and adding a dissociative subtype (Möller et al., 2015). Current diagnostic criteria group symptoms into four clusters: re-experiencing, avoidance, negative changes in mood and cognition, and hyperarousal (Monson et al., 2009; O'Toole et al., 2020; Roth et al., 2016). Veterans often present across multiple clusters simultaneously, which contributes to the complexity of assessment and treatment (Maercker et al., 2013; Steenkamp & Litz, 2013).

The complexity of PTSD has important implications for treatment. Veterans who have experienced combat trauma may live with overlapping symptoms, including recurrent reminders of trauma, extreme avoidance, and mood disturbances. These symptoms are compounded by physiological stress responses, which can exacerbate hypervigilance and arousal (Ehlers & Clark, 2000; Yehuda, 2002). Many veterans also remain reluctant to seek psychological care, with stigma and cultural attitudes leading some to self-medicate with alcohol or other substances instead of accessing professional support (Brenner et al., 2009; Troyanskaya et al., 2015). Such patterns highlight the gap between diagnostic clarity and the lived experience of PTSD, underlining the need for treatment models that are not only evidence-based but also flexible, patient-centred, and responsive to veterans' realities (Berntsen et al., 2012; DiMauro et al., 2014).

Orthodox Treatments

The complex symptomatology of PTSD means that treatment often requires a combination of psychological and pharmaceutical approaches. First-line trauma-focused therapies such as CBT, CPT, and EMDR remain the most widely prescribed psychological interventions and have been shown to bring clinical improvement for around half of veterans who undertake them (Benedek et al., 2009; Cloitre, 2009; Reisman, 2016; Van der Kolk & Najavits, 2013). Yet dropout rates remain high, with up to 30% of veterans discontinuing treatment due to the emotional difficulty of confronting traumatic content, challenges in building trust with therapists, and the limited durability of symptom relief (Doukas et al., 2014; Levi et al., 2016).

Pharmacological interventions are also commonly prescribed, with SSRIs and SNRIs representing the most frequently used classes (Stein et al., 2009; Jeffreys, 2009). While some veterans report partial relief of symptoms such as anxiety or depression, overall response rates are modest, with many requiring complex combinations of medications to target hyperarousal, avoidance, and mood disturbance (Bernardy et al., 2012; MacManus et al., 2012; Sauvé & Stahl, 2019). Research continues to suggest that medication alone rarely provides sufficient symptom management, particularly for veterans with multiple comorbidities (Frueh et al., 2005; Jablonski et al., 2015).

Taken together, orthodox treatments offer benefits for many but fall short of delivering consistent and long-lasting relief across the veteran population. Their limitations, high dropout rates, partial efficacy, and difficulty addressing the full spectrum of PTSD symptoms, underscore the pressing need for adjunctive and innovative approaches (Steenkamp et al., 2020; Strauss et al., 2011). This recognition has contributed to growing interest in alternatives, with approximately 40% of veterans exploring holistic or complementary practices to alleviate symptoms such as anxiety, depression, and hyperarousal (Wahbeh et al., 2014). These trends point to the importance of broadening the range of interventions available, including the systematic consideration of exercise as a therapeutic adjunct.

Unorthodox Therapies

Alongside conventional treatments, many veterans with PTSD have explored alternative or unorthodox therapies. These include the controlled use of MDMA, CBD, and high-THC cannabis, which have shown promise in alleviating symptoms such as anxiety, depression, and hyperarousal (Forsythe & Boileau, 2021; Strauss et al., 2011; Wahbeh et al., 2014; Mitchell et al., 2021; Varker et al., 2021). However, these substances may also disrupt REM sleep, which plays a critical role in processing traumatic experiences (Loflin et al., 2017; O'Brien et al., 2021; Kolla et al., 2022). Individual variation in response is significant, and further research is required to understand the long-term impact on veterans' health and functioning (Geldenhuys et al., 2022).

Other approaches emphasise psychological and holistic practices. Mindfulness, meditation, guided imagery, relaxation techniques, and deep breathing exercises have all been reported to support coping and emotional regulation in veterans with PTSD (Forsythe & Boileau, 2021; Strauss et al., 2011; Wahbeh et al., 2014). Similarly, yoga and other naturopathic practices have been associated with improvements in holistic well-being and may serve as useful complements to established therapies. These approaches illustrate the importance of broadening the toolkit available to veterans, even if they are not yet established as first-line treatments.

Survey evidence indicates that roughly 40% of veterans with PTSD have experimented with alternative or holistic medicine to alleviate symptoms (Wahbeh et al., 2014). While such therapies can be beneficial for some, they often lack the robust empirical foundation needed to replace evidence-based care. Their role, therefore, should be viewed as supplementary rather than primary.

At the same time, the limitations of orthodox approaches, including dropout rates in psychotherapy, the finite duration of relief from medications, and the frequent need for polypharmacy, create space for veterans to seek additional options (Cloitre, 2009; Doukas et al., 2014; Levi et al., 2016; Stein et al., 2009). The growing interest in unorthodox therapies underscores a wider imperative: to investigate innovative, patient-centred interventions that can be integrated safely and effectively alongside existing treatments. Among these, physical exercise offers a particularly promising pathway.

Moving Exercise from an Unorthodox to an Orthodox Treatment

The evidence presented across this monograph highlights a clear deficit in the way exercise has traditionally been considered in PTSD treatment. Despite growing recognition, physical activity remains on the margins of orthodox approaches, yet research increasingly suggests that it offers substantial potential benefits. Exercise has been shown to alleviate a range of PTSD symptoms while also improving general physical and mental health (Broman-Fulks et al., 2004; Caddick & Smith, 2014, 2018; Foote et al., 2015).

Different modes of exercise appear to provide distinct advantages. Aerobic activities such as running, swimming, and walking have been associated with reductions in anxiety, depression, hyperarousal, and improved sleep quality (Hegberg et al., 2019; Smith & Merwin, 2021). Resistance training and other anaerobic activities have demonstrated benefits for muscle strength and emotional regulation, particularly in reducing anger and stress reactivity (Hegberg et al., 2019; Smith & Merwin, 2021). Flexibility-based practices such as yoga or Pilates have been linked to reduced tension and stress (Michailidis et al., 2013; Whitworth & Ciccolo, 2016), while functional and movement-based activities, including Tai chi, have been shown to foster confidence, resilience, and overall fitness (Mobbs & Bonanno, 2018; Hegberg et al., 2019). Taken together, these findings suggest that exercise can provide multidimensional benefits that parallel, and in some cases exceed, those of more established therapies.

It is important to acknowledge, however, that exercise is not a universal remedy. Some veterans may encounter barriers such as accessibility, stigma, or the risk of triggering traumatic memories (Hudetz et al., 2010; Hegberg et al., 2019). Responses to exercise are also highly individual, emphasising the need for flexibility in prescribing and supporting its use (Hopkins et al., 2009; Caddick & Smith, 2018). Nonetheless, the balance of evidence suggests that the advantages far outweigh the limitations.

As interest in alternative and complementary therapies grows, exercise stands out as uniquely positioned to bridge the gap between orthodox and unorthodox treatment modalities. Its benefits are supported by a growing evidence base, and it offers veterans an accessible, empowering, and cost-effective means of improving both physical and psychological health (Caddick et al., 2015; Hegberg et al., 2019). Integrating structured physical activity into treatment plans has the potential to transform PTSD care, moving exercise from an unorthodox supplement to a recognised prescription alongside psychological and pharmaceutical interventions.

Results

This monograph represents a departure from traditional approaches by adopting an interdisciplinary stance, seeking to understand how military veterans respond to existing PTSD treatments and to explore the potential role of exercise as a complementary modality. Rather than attempting to replicate the strict conditions of a randomised controlled trial, which was neither feasible nor ethical in this context, the research embraced a hybrid design. The aim was to examine exercise patterns and habits, assess veterans' perceptions of its utility in managing symptoms, and explore how physical activity might contribute to overall well-being when combined with conventional therapies.

The findings derive from three interconnected studies: an autoethnography, a series of interviews, and an online survey. Taken together, these strands provided a multifaceted picture of the relationship between exercise and PTSD, illuminating both the opportunities and challenges of integrating physical activity into treatment pathways. Each strand contributed unique insights: the autoethnography foregrounded lived experience, the interviews captured veterans' voices and perspectives, and the survey offered a broader snapshot of exercise patterns and their reported impact.

These results inform the central argument of this monograph: that exercise can play a meaningful role in the recovery journeys of veterans with PTSD, not as a replacement for orthodox therapies, but as a valuable addition to them. The implications extend beyond individual experiences, offering lessons for medical professionals, veteran support organisations, and policymakers about the importance of flexible, patient-centred treatment strategies.

The findings derive from three interconnected studies: an autoethnography, a series of interviews, and an online survey. The autoethnography provided a foundation, offering insight into lived experience, while the interviews and survey expanded this perspective with voices from across the veteran community.

Autoethnography

The first strand of this research drew on autoethnography to explore the role of exercise in my own experience of PTSD. Earlier attempts to manage symptoms through running, cycling and weightlifting had little effect, which led me to experiment with CrossFit®. This approach became a lens through which I examined the intersection of lived experience and psychological theory. In particular, the principles of Self-Determination Theory (SDT), namely autonomy, competence and relatedness, provided a framework for understanding how exercise could foster transformation and resilience (Deci & Ryan, 1985; Ryan, 2009; Ryan et al., 2019).

Autonomy was evident in the decision to pursue CrossFit® as a self-directed strategy during a period of emotional turmoil and isolation. In line with SDT, this act represented a reclaiming of personal agency by engaging in activities that reflected my own values and needs (Deci & Ryan, 1985; Ryan & Deci, 2000; Claudino et al., 2018). Competence also emerged as a central theme. CrossFit® provided an outlet for converting distress into mastery and growth, illustrating how physical training can support emotional resilience and empowerment (Caddick & Smith, 2014; Ryan et al., 2012). Finally, relatedness was embodied in the strong bonds developed within the CrossFit® community, where the mutual encouragement of peers offered emotional support and became an important resource for healing.

Taken together, these experiences highlight the potential of exercise environments such as CrossFit® to facilitate more than just physical gains. They can create spaces where autonomy, competence, and relatedness intersect to support psychological well-being and post-traumatic growth. While these findings are personal, they illustrate how theoretical frameworks can illuminate lived experience and provide insights that extend to wider veteran populations. The narrative demonstrates that physical exercise can act as a catalyst for self-transformation, complementing orthodox treatments by offering agency, resilience, and a sense of belonging (Deci & Ryan, 1985; Ryan et al., 2019).

These insights also point towards broader implications. They show how exercise can help veterans reclaim control in contexts where traditional treatments may feel disempowering. They also highlight the value of community-based approaches, where social bonds and shared endeavour can act as protective factors against isolation and despair. While rooted in one individual's experience, the findings resonate with themes expressed by many veterans, offering a foundation for future exploration of exercise as a structured therapeutic intervention.

Interviews

The interviews with six veterans provided insight into how physical exercise shaped their lives before and after a PTSD diagnosis, and how it continues to function as a tool for managing symptoms. All participants had a long history of physical activity, consistent with the culture and expectations of military service. From an early age, exercise was woven into their identities, fostering discipline, resilience, and a sense of purpose. This strong foundation of physical engagement meant that when PTSD symptoms emerged later in life, exercise was already positioned as a familiar and trusted strategy for coping (Paluska & Schwenk, 2000; Teixeira et al., 2012; Ashdown-Franks et al., 2019; Hegberg et al., 2019).

Participants described clear therapeutic benefits when using exercise to manage PTSD symptoms. Activities such as swimming, cycling, yoga and running were credited with reducing stress, alleviating intrusive thoughts and providing temporary relief from the burden of trauma. The physiological release that came from exertion, including the effect of endorphins, was often experienced as a reset, reducing both the frequency and intensity of episodes (Björkman & Ekblom, 2022; Lee et al., 2022). These accounts reinforced a theme found in the wider literature: that exercise can function as an important adjunctive treatment by creating space for calm, clarity, and recovery.

Beyond symptom relief, exercise promoted wider behavioural change. Veterans described establishing structured routines, embracing discipline and perseverance, and noticing improvements in their physical capability alongside their mental state. Exercise was understood not simply as activity but as a form of self-care, a way to regain control and actively participate in recovery. This sense of agency reflected findings that exercise can foster empowerment and resilience, helping individuals move beyond passivity in their treatment journeys (Mikkelsen et al., 2017; Whitworth et al., 2017).

A final theme emerged in the participants' comparison between exercise and traditional treatments such as cognitive-behavioural therapy or medication. While acknowledging the place of these orthodox approaches, many expressed a preference for exercise, describing it as more holistic, personally fulfilling, and empowering. The mind-body connection created through physical activity was valued as an alternative way of processing distress, reinforcing the idea that effective treatment is not only about symptom reduction but also about enabling veterans to feel ownership of their healing (Lastuka & Cottingham, 2016; Oppizzi & Umberger, 2018).

Taken together, the interviews underscored four interconnected themes: the deep significance of pre-diagnosis activity, the clear symptom relief experienced through exercise, the behavioural transformations fostered after diagnosis, and the preference for exercise as a holistic alternative or complement to standard treatments. These findings reveal the potential of physical activity to bridge gaps left by orthodox interventions, highlighting the need for patient-centred strategies that accommodate individual preferences and lived experiences. Importantly, they also point towards the value of recognising exercise as a legitimate therapeutic pathway within formal care settings for veterans with PTSD.

Survey

The survey findings added breadth to the insights from the autoethnography and interviews by capturing patterns across a larger group of veterans. Analysis of responses to a 27-item questionnaire showed that participants reported clear preferences for different forms of exercise, as well as barriers to engagement. Diversity in exercise choices emerged as a consistent theme. While aerobic activity such as running, swimming and cycling was the most popular, many also favoured anaerobic training, flexibility-based exercise, or functional movement. This reinforces evidence that multiple modalities can support recovery from PTSD and highlights the importance of tailoring interventions to individual needs (Hegberg et al., 2019; Lopes-Silva et al., 2018; Asmundson et al., 2013; Mikkelsen et al., 2017).

Most participants rejected the idea that exercise worsens symptoms. Instead, they identified benefits in managing stress, improving sleep, reducing anxiety, and alleviating depression. These views echo existing research that positions exercise as a holistic form of PTSD management rather than a source of risk (Caddick & Smith, 2014; Shirazipour et al., 2017; Michailidis et al., 2013; Oppizzi & Umberger, 2018). At the same time, some veterans reported difficulties maintaining routines, with avoidance behaviours, traumatic memories or side effects from medication interfering with adherence. This variability reflects the complex interaction between PTSD symptoms and exercise engagement (Rosenbaum et al., 2015; Thompson-Hollands et al., 2021; Crombie et al., 2023; Begin et al., 2019).

The survey also revealed differences in satisfaction with existing treatment approaches. While some were content with orthodox care, others expressed frustration with limited progress and turned to exercise for greater empowerment and control. A preference for personalised programmes emerged, though not all participants sought the same level of tailoring. This tension between structured interventions and individual choice underscores the need for flexibility and patient-centred planning (Klimek et al., 2018; Björkman & Ekblom, 2022).

Conceptual analysis of open responses reinforced these patterns. Some veterans described negative effects such as heightened anxiety, noise sensitivity, migraines or nausea, indicating that exercise can sometimes trigger symptoms or clash with existing treatments (Goldstein et al., 2018; Walker et al., 2016). However, the majority reported either no adverse effects or clear benefits, identifying themes of empowerment, revitalisation, and calm. These findings align with research showing that physical activity can contribute to self-efficacy and psychological resilience when appropriately supported (Ashdown-Franks et al., 2019; Patki et al., 2014; Adams et al., 2020).

Taken together, the survey highlights the potential of structured exercise to serve as a valuable complement to orthodox treatments. It confirms that veterans' preferences are diverse, that engagement is sometimes fragile, and that outcomes are shaped by both individual histories and the contexts in which exercise takes place. These insights provide a platform for designing interventions that are flexible, patient-led, and integrated into broader care plans for veterans with PTSD. They also establish the link between lived experience and policy relevance, setting the stage for the implications and recommendations that follow.

Implications

This monograph carries significance for both scholarship and practice because it demonstrates how exercise can play a substantial role in enhancing the well-being of veterans with PTSD. By presenting exercise as a holistic and empowering approach, it challenges the limitations of conventional treatments and promotes a patient-centred model of care. The findings suggest that exercise can serve as a supplementary therapy, providing veterans with a renewed sense of control, resilience, and improved mental health (Nicholson & McLoughlin, 2019).

The implications extend beyond the individual veteran. They should resonate with stakeholders across the healthcare and veteran-support landscape, including the Ministry of Defence, NHS England, medical professionals, therapists, veteran charities such as the British Legion, Help for Heroes, and Combat Stress, as well as policymakers who shape the delivery of services. For these groups, the findings highlight a practical opportunity: to embed structured physical exercise as a legitimate and beneficial element of PTSD treatment (Caddick & Smith, 2014; Daffey-Moore, 2020; Hegberg et al., 2019).

Policy change is central to this discussion. Initiatives such as Op COURAGE, the Veterans' Mental Health Transition, Intervention and Liaison Service, and the High-Intensity Service already provide valuable support to veterans and their families. Yet these schemes could be enriched by the systematic inclusion of exercise-based programmes alongside orthodox therapies (Finnegan et al., 2025; Shirazipour et al., 2017). Recognising exercise as a prescribed option, delivered in a structured and supported way, would strengthen the effectiveness of existing services and create more flexible, patient-focused treatment pathways.

Funding and training will be crucial to this shift. The UK government, through the NHS and the Ministry of Defence, should allocate resources to train occupational health specialists and therapists in the use of exercise as a therapeutic intervention. General practitioners and service providers within Op COURAGE could then prescribe exercise alongside standard treatment plans, with regular reviews to evaluate its impact on symptoms. Additional investment through the Armed Forces Covenant and collaboration with local authorities would help embed exercise programmes within the wider veteran community (Crombie et al., 2023).

Practical implementation also requires partnership with existing organisations. Veterans could be guided towards local opportunities by designated Armed Forces Champions, whose remit already includes connecting former service members with community resources. Help for Heroes hubs provide another avenue, offering structured activities such as walking groups, archery, cycling, and climbing, all of which align with the findings of this research and can foster both physical and social recovery (Whitworth et al., 2017). Similarly, animal-assisted interventions, such as those facilitated by Hounds for Heroes and Veterans with Dogs, highlight how engagement in physical activity and care routines can ease isolation, provide companionship, and reduce anxiety.

The evidence also points to the need for veterans to make exercise a consistent part of their daily lives. Routine transforms physical activity from a sporadic coping mechanism into a sustained habit that supports long-term well-being. This is not without challenges: adherence is often difficult, and routines must be varied, enjoyable, and sensitive to individual needs (Oppizzi & Umberger, 2018). Trainers and facilitators therefore require specialist knowledge of PTSD in order to design appropriate programmes. Online platforms could expand access, allowing veterans to participate from home while receiving guidance tailored to their condition (Rosenbaum et al., 2015).

Taken together, the implications of this monograph emphasise that exercise is not a replacement for orthodox therapies but a powerful complement to them. Integrating physical activity into PTSD care offers a patient-centred model that is flexible, empowering, and grounded in lived experience. The challenge for policymakers, clinicians, and support organisations is to ensure that veterans can access programmes that are structured, supported, and sustainable, enabling exercise to fulfil its potential as part of a comprehensive approach to recovery.

Limitations of Monograph

This monograph contributes to the broader body of research on whether physical exercise can be an alternative or complementary therapeutic method for military veterans with PTSD. However, several limitations must be acknowledged. A key constraint was the small sample sizes across the empirical studies. The interview-based study involved only six participants, and the survey included nineteen. Such limited numbers inevitably reduce statistical power and restrict the extent to which the findings can be generalised. A larger cohort, closer to 50 participants, would have enhanced both the reliability and transferability of results, enabling a more detailed exploration of the relationship between exercise and PTSD symptomology (Creswell, 2009).

The research design also imposed certain constraints. The work was conducted within a relatively short timeframe, which precluded a longitudinal approach. A longer-term study would have allowed the tracking of veterans' experiences over time, providing insight into whether the benefits of exercise persist or evolve. Such designs would also offer a richer understanding of the dynamic nature of PTSD and the long-term role of physical activity in symptom management and overall well-being (Yehuda, 2002).

The application of Self-Determination Theory (SDT) in the autoethnography carried its own limitations. While SDT offered a valuable framework for understanding motivation, it relied heavily on subjective narrative and interpretation, which introduces the risk of bias. Moreover, the focus on CrossFit® created a context-specific lens that may not generalise to other forms of exercise or broader veteran populations. SDT itself does not establish causal relationships, and reliance on self-report data carries the potential for social desirability bias. Finally, the emphasis on positive aspects of motivation and behaviour risks underrepresenting negative or ambivalent experiences.

Another important limitation is that the findings cannot be generalised to the entire population of veterans with PTSD. Recruitment through specific channels may have introduced selection bias, and the relatively small, self-selecting group of participants may not represent the diversity of the wider veteran community. Future studies would benefit from broader recruitment strategies, random sampling where possible, and larger, more diverse cohorts to capture a fuller spectrum of experiences (Creswell, 2009).

A further consideration is the positionality of the researcher. As a veteran diagnosed with PTSD, my lived experience was both a strength and a potential source of bias. While I sought to mitigate this through independent data analysis, peer review, and adherence to ethical standards, it remains important to recognise that my perspective shaped the framing and interpretation of the research. This dual role highlights the need for reflexivity and transparency when combining personal narrative with academic analysis (Finlay, 2002).

In conclusion, the limitations of this monograph, including small sample sizes, design constraints, reliance on subjective frameworks, and potential researcher bias, underscore the need for continued investigation.

Future research should pursue larger and more diverse samples, employ longitudinal and controlled designs, and further explore which exercise modalities are most effective for veterans with PTSD. Yet despite these limitations, the contribution of this monograph is significant. By combining lived experience with systematic inquiry, it demonstrates the potential of physical exercise to enhance recovery and well-being, not as a replacement for orthodox therapies but as a powerful complement to them. In doing so, it advances both scholarship and practice, and most importantly, it gives voice to the experiences of veterans whose struggles are too often marginalised.

Future Research

The overarching aim of this monograph was to investigate the efficacy of physical exercise as a treatment method for military veterans with PTSD. The findings presented here add important insight to the wider body of research on the role of exercise in PTSD management. Building upon the results from Chaps. 4 and 5, and drawing in particular from the autoethnography, the next step is to develop a longitudinal CrossFit® intervention that provides a sustained and systematic assessment of exercise in supporting recovery. This is timely work: too many veterans continue to fall through the gaps of existing provision, highlighting the urgent need for approaches that are flexible, accessible, and grounded in lived experience.

I propose implementing a rolling 12-week CrossFit® intervention over a 24-month period. CrossFit® is particularly suited to this context because it combines aerobic activity, strength training, and flexibility work, while its scalability allows participants of different fitness levels to engage meaningfully. The programme's emphasis on functional movement and adaptability ensures that veterans with varied needs can participate safely and effectively. This represents a pioneering intervention, as no previous study has examined a longitudinal CrossFit® Programme in a veteran PTSD population.

The design incorporates diverse exercise modalities to address both physical and psychological aspects of recovery. Aerobic activities such as running, rowing, and cycling will aim to enhance endurance and mood, reducing PTSD symptomology. Strength training will focus on building capability and confidence, while flexibility and mobility work will support relaxation and joint health. Together, these components provide a holistic intervention designed to promote resilience, well-being, and long-term adherence.

Systematic data collection will be central. Participants will undergo regular assessments of PTSD symptoms, physical fitness, and psychological well-being, with data gathered before and after each 12-week cycle. Quantitative measures will capture measurable change, while qualitative feedback will ensure that veterans' voices remain central to the analysis. This mixed-methods approach provides both scientific robustness and patient-centred depth, enabling outcomes that are credible to clinicians and meaningful to veterans.

This proposed CrossFit® intervention represents an extension of the current research and an important step in strengthening the evidence base for exercise as a complementary treatment for PTSD. If successful, it has the potential not only to transform care practices for veterans but also to inform national provision by integrating exercise into initiatives such as Op COURAGE, the NHS Veterans' Mental Health Services, and Help for Heroes hubs. In doing so, it can contribute to policy debates about patient-centred treatment, the role of non-orthodox therapies within mainstream care, and the long-term sustainability of mental health provision for veterans.

Future research should also expand beyond CrossFit®, comparing different exercise modalities and exploring their effectiveness across diverse veteran populations. Such comparative work will be critical in refining evidence-based recommendations for clinical practice and shaping policy, ensuring that physical exercise becomes a recognised and sustainable element of PTSD care.

Final Declaration

Some monographs are written as personal reflections, helping the author make sense of their own journey. Others serve primarily to consolidate the state of knowledge or to advance scientific understanding for application in health, education, or policy. This monograph seeks to achieve all of these, but it also aims to provide something more: hope.

It was born out of struggle, not only my own but also that of the veterans who participated in this research. Together, we contributed to this work in the hope of building a brighter future. In this sense, the monograph is not mine alone. It is for the brothers and sisters I served alongside, for their families, and for the wider community of veterans living with PTSD.

The work continues a long line of efforts to bring PTSD out of denial, to deepen understanding of its complex aetiology, and to search for effective ways of treating it. By highlighting the role of physical exercise as a complementary pathway to recovery, it challenges conventional approaches and points to new opportunities for practice and policy.

If this monograph achieves anything, I hope it is to make a difference—in the lives of veterans, in the services that support them, and in the way society understands and responds to PTSD.

References

Adams, R. E., Boscarino, J. A., & Galea, S. (2020). Physical activity, distress, and coping in trauma-exposed adults. *American Journal of Preventive Medicine, 58*(2), 216–224.

Ashdown-Franks, G., Firth, J., Carney, R., Carvalho, A. F., Hallgren, M., Koyanagi, A., & Stubbs, B. (2019). Exercise as medicine for mental and substance use disorders: A meta-review of benefits and harms. *British Journal of Sports Medicine, 54*(19), 1144–1153.

Asmundson, G. J. G., Fetzner, M. G., DeBoer, L. B., Powers, M. B., Otto, M. W., & Smits, J. A. J. (2013). Let's get physical: A contemporary review of the anxiolytic effects of exercise for anxiety and its disorders. *Depression and Anxiety, 30*(4), 362–373.

Begin, M. E., Deschênes, S. S., & Blais, R. K. (2019). Satisfaction with PTSD care and treatment preferences among veterans. *Psychological Services, 16*(4), 557–565.

Benedek, D. M., Friedman, M. J., Zatzick, D., & Ursano, R. J. (2009). Guideline-concordant acute stress disorder and PTSD treatment. *Psychiatric Annals, 39*(6), 345–354.

Bernardy, N. C., Friedman, M. J., Jensen, S. E., Zegers, A., & Zatzick, D. (2012). Pharmacotherapy for posttraumatic stress disorder in military and veteran populations. *Journal of Clinical Psychiatry, 73*(10), 1284–1290.

Berntsen, D., Johannessen, K. B., Thomsen, Y. D., Bertelsen, M., Hoyle, R. H., & Rubin, D. C. (2012). Peacekeepers' memories of war: A field study of the impact of traumatic stress reactions on everyday memories. *Journal of Behaviour Therapy and Experimental Psychiatry, 43*(1), 821–829.

Björkman, F., & Ekblom, Ö. (2022). Physical activity in the treatment of PTSD: Opportunities and barriers. *European Journal of Psychotraumatology, 13*(1), 205–218.

Brenner, L. A., Vanderploeg, R. D., & Terrio, H. (2009). Assessment and treatment of individuals with history of traumatic brain injury and post-traumatic stress disorder: A clinical review. *Journal of Head Trauma Rehabilitation, 24*(6), 410–419.

Broman-Fulks, J. J., Berman, M. E., Rabian, B. A., & Webster, M. J. (2004). Effects of aerobic exercise on anxiety sensitivity. *Behaviour Research and Therapy, 42*(2), 125–136.

Caddick, N., Phoenix, C., & Smith, B. (2015). Collective stories of exercise in the military: A social identity approach to understanding veterans' experiences. *Qualitative Research in Sport, Exercise and Health, 7*(1), 42–61.

Caddick, N., & Smith, B. (2014). The impact of sport and physical activity on the lives of military veterans with PTSD. *Psychology of Sport and Exercise, 15*(1), 9–18.

Caddick, N., & Smith, B. (2018). Exercise as a coping resource for military veterans with PTSD. *Qualitative Health Research, 28*(3), 1–13.

Claudino, J. G., Gabbett, T. J., Bourgeois, F., Souza, H. D. S., Miranda, R. C., Mezêncio, B., ... & Serrão, J. C. (2018). CrossFit® training strategies and psycho-behavioural effects. *Sports Medicine, 48*(2), 1–23.

Cloitre, M. (2009). Effective psychotherapies for posttraumatic stress disorder: A review and critique. *CNS Spectrums, 14*(1), 32–43.

Connell, J. (2016). A cultural history of post-traumatic stress disorder. *Cultural Sociology, 10*(4), 483–497.

Creswell, J. W. (2009). *Research design: Qualitative, quantitative, and mixed methods approaches* (3rd ed.). Sage.

Crombie, D., Smith, L., & Beck, K. (2023). Exercise participation, sleep, and mood in veterans receiving mental health care. *Mental Health and Physical Activity, 24*, 100–112.

Daffey-Moore, J. (2020). Embedding exercise within NHS veteran services. *Journal of the Royal Army Medical Corps, 166*(3), 230–233.

Deci, E. L., & Ryan, R. M. (1985). *Intrinsic motivation and self-determination in human behaviour*. Plenum.

DiMauro, J., Renshaw, K. D., Smith, C. V., & Vogt, D. S. (2014). Stigma and barriers to care among veterans with PTSD. *Psychological Services, 11*(1), 54–64.

Doukas, A., Batten, S. V., & Harvey, M. (2014). Dropout from PTSD psychotherapy in veterans: A systematic review. *Journal of Traumatic Stress, 27*(6), 563–570.

Dyball, D., Jones, N., Fear, N. T., & Wessely, S. (2022). Post-traumatic stress disorder symptoms in UK combat-injured personnel after deployment. *Occupational Medicine, 72*(4), 255–262.

Ehlers, A., & Clark, D. M. (2000). A cognitive model of posttraumatic stress disorder. *Behaviour Research and Therapy, 38*(4), 319–345.

Finlay, L. (2002). Negotiating the swamp: The opportunity and challenge of reflexivity in research practice. *Qualitative Research, 2*(2), 209–230.

Finnegan, A., Greenberg, N., & Jones, N. (2025). Op COURAGE: Service development and evaluation in veteran mental health. *BMJ Military Health, 171*(1), 10–15.

Foote, D. C., Piazza, J. R., & Sonnega, A. (2015). Exercise as an adjunctive treatment for PTSD: A narrative review. *Journal of Clinical Psychology in Medical Settings, 22*(3), 213–222.

Forsythe, L., & Boileau, I. (2021). Psychedelics and cannabinoids in PTSD: Promise and pitfalls. *Current Opinion in Psychology, 38*, 72–77.

Frueh, B. C., Grubaugh, A. L., Elhai, J. D., & Buckley, T. C. (2005). US Department of Veterans Affairs PTSD treatment practices and outcomes. *International Journal of Psychiatry in Medicine, 35*(3), 241–250.

Geldenhuys, W., Sorsdahl, K., & Stein, D. J. (2022). Long-term health effects of cannabinoid use in PTSD. *Progress in Neuro-Psychopharmacology and Biological Psychiatry, 112*, 110–120.

Goldstein, E., Topitzes, J., Brown, R. L., & Barrett, B. (2018). Traumatic stress, exercise, and clinical considerations: A narrative review. *Journal of Clinical Medicine, 7*(4), 89–102.

Grillon, C., & Morgan, C. A. (1999). Fear-potentiated startle in Vietnam veterans with PTSD. *Biological Psychiatry, 45*(4), 405–417.

Hegberg, N. J., Hayes, J. P., & Hayes, S. M. (2019). Exercise intervention in PTSD: A narrative review and rationale. *Frontiers in Psychiatry, 10*, 133.

Hopkins, W. G., Marshall, S. W., Batterham, A. M., & Hanin, J. (2009). Progressive statistics for studies in sports medicine and exercise science. *Medicine & Science in Sports & Exercise, 41*(1), 3–13.

Hudetz, J. A., Warltier, D. C., & Pagel, P. S. (2010). Heterogeneous response to PTSD treatments: Mechanistic considerations. *Journal of Neuropsychiatry and Clinical Neurosciences, 22*(2), 123–128.

Jablonski, M., Pugh, M. J. V., & Janak, J. C. (2015). Polypharmacy and outcomes in veterans with PTSD. *CNS Drugs, 29*(10), 847–857.

Jeffreys, M. (2009). Pharmacotherapy for posttraumatic stress disorder: Evidence-based practice. *Journal of Clinical Psychiatry, 70*(Suppl 2), 16–22.

Karlin, B. E., Ruzek, J. I., Chard, K. M., Eftekhari, A., Monson, C. M., Hembree, E. A., ... & Foa, E. B. (2010). Dissemination of evidence-based psychotherapies for posttraumatic stress disorder in the Veterans Health Administration. *Psychological Services, 7*(4), 354–365.

Klimek, L., Bergmann, K. C., & Biedermann, T. (2018). Triggers and safety considerations for exercise in trauma-exposed populations. *Allergy, 73*(12), 2474–2486.

Kolla, B. P., Mansukhani, M. P., & Bostwick, J. M. (2022). Cannabis and sleep: Implications for PTSD. *Current Psychiatry Reports, 24*(2), 45–54.

Lastuka, A., & Cottingham, M. (2016). The effect of adaptive sport programmes on veterans' well-being. *Disability and Health Journal, 9*(2), 281–288.

Lee, D., Thomas, S. A., & Taylor, G. (2022). Physical activity and mental health outcomes among veterans: A systematic review. *Military Medicine, 187*(5–6), e585–e593.

Leightley, D., Puddephatt, J.-A., Jones, N., Mahmoodi, T., Field, M., & Fear, N. T. (2019). Mental health prevalence in UK Armed Forces veterans. *European Journal of Psychotraumatology, 10*(1), 154–167.

Levi, O., Horesh, D., & Ginzburg, K. (2016). Reasons for dropout from trauma-focused therapies: Patients' perspectives. *Psychological Trauma: Theory, Research, Practice, and Policy, 8*(6), 702–711.

Loflin, M. J. E., Earleywine, M., & Bonn-Miller, M. O. (2017). Cannabinoids and sleep architecture in PTSD. *Psychology of Addictive Behaviours, 31*(6), 745–753.

Lopes-Silva, J. P., Dos Santos, J. V., & Loturco, I. (2018). High-intensity training and stress regulation in combat veterans. *Frontiers in Physiology, 9*, 1920.

MacManus, D., Wessely, S., & Fear, N. T. (2012). Prescribing patterns for PTSD in the UK Armed Forces. *BMJ Open, 2*(6), e001571.

Maercker, A., Brewin, C. R., Bryant, R. A., Cloitre, M., Van Ommeren, M., Jones, L. M., ... & Reed, G. M. (2013). Diagnosis of PTSD and complex PTSD in ICD-11: Clinical implications. *World Psychiatry, 12*(3), 198–206.

Michailidis, Y., Vagenas, G., & Koutedakis, Y. (2013). The effect of relaxation techniques and yoga on stress reduction. *Complementary Therapies in Medicine, 21*(6), 648–655.

Mikkelsen, K., Stojanovska, L., Polenakovic, M., Bosevski, M., & Apostolopoulos, V. (2017). Exercise and mental health. *Maturitas, 106*, 48–56.

Mitchell, J. M., Bogenschutz, M., Lilienstein, A., Harrison, C., Kleiman, S., Parker-Guilbert, K., ... & Doblin, R. (2021). MDMA-assisted therapy for severe PTSD: A randomised, double-blind, placebo-controlled Phase 3 study. *Nature Medicine, 27*(6), 1025–1033.

Mobbs, M. C., & Bonanno, G. A. (2018). Beyond war and PTSD: The positive psychology of military service. *American Psychologist, 73*(5), 644–654.

Möller, H.-J., Bandelow, B., Volz, H.-P., Barnikol, U. B., Seifritz, E., & Kasper, S. (2015). The relevance of DSM-5 for psychiatric diagnoses. *International Journal of Psychiatry in Clinical Practice, 19*(1), 2–8.

Monson, C. M., Gradus, J. L., Young-Xu, Y., & Schnurr, P. P. (2009). The role of PTSD symptom clusters and functioning. *Journal of Anxiety Disorders, 23*(2), 223–230.

Nicholson, E., & McLoughlin, D. (2019). Exercise referral schemes and mental health outcomes: A narrative review. *Irish Journal of Medical Science, 188*(2), 527–534.

O'Brien, L. M., Stocker, R. P., & Manber, R. (2021). Sleep, trauma, and pharmacological treatment. *Sleep Medicine Reviews, 55*, 101–108.

O'Toole, B. I., Outram, S., Catts, S. V., & Pierse, K. R. (2020). PTSD symptom structure in veterans: An epidemiological approach. *Journal of Affective Disorders, 266*, 282–289.

Oppizzi, L. M., & Umberger, R. (2018). The effect of physical activity on sleep quality, mood, and wellbeing in veterans. *Journal of Clinical Sleep Medicine, 14*(4), 649–658.

Paluska, S. A., & Schwenk, T. L. (2000). Physical activity and mental health: Current concepts and applications. *Sports Medicine, 29*(3), 167–180.

Patki, G., Solanki, N., & Salim, S. (2014). Exercise as a therapeutic intervention in stress-induced psychiatric disorders. *Neuropharmacology, 77*, 232–247.

Reisman, M. (2016). PTSD treatment update. *Primary Care Companion for CNS Disorders, 18*(6), 1–9.

Rosenbaum, S., Tiedemann, A., Ward, P. B., & Curtis, J. (2015). Barriers to exercise among people with mental illness. *BMC Psychiatry, 15*, 52.

Rosenfeld, J. V., McFarlane, A. C., Bragge, P., & Armfield, N. R. (2013). Health outcomes of recent UK military operations: Combat injury and mental health. *Journal of Military and Veterans' Health, 21*(4), 6–14.

Roth, T. L., Liberzon, I., & Milad, M. R. (2016). Neurobiology of PTSD: From brain circuits to treatment. *Neuropsychopharmacology, 41*(1), 297–319.

Ryan, R. M. (2009). Self-determination theory and well-being. *Social and Personality Psychology Compass, 3*(1), 1–18.

Ryan, R. M., & Deci, E. L. (2000). Self-determination theory and the facilitation of intrinsic motivation, social development, and well-being. *American Psychologist, 55*(1), 68–78.

Ryan, R. M., Deci, E. L., Vansteenkiste, M., & Soenens, B. (2019). Building a science of motivated persons: Self-determination theory's empirical approach to human experience and the regulation of behaviour. *Motivation Science, 5*(2), 97–110.

Ryan, R. M., Huta, V., & Deci, E. L. (2012). Living well: A self-determination theory perspective on eudaimonia. *Journal of Happiness Studies, 13*(1), 109–119.

Sauvé, G., & Stahl, S. M. (2019). Pharmacotherapy pearls in PTSD: Practical clinical considerations. *CNS Spectrums, 24*(2), 245–253.

Shirazipour, C. H., Evans, M. B., & Spence, J. C. (2017). Exploring the impact of physical activity on veterans with PTSD. *Psychology of Sport and Exercise, 30*, 179–188.

Smith, B., & Merwin, R. M. (2021). Resistance training and affect regulation in PTSD. *Frontiers in Psychology, 12*, 640–649.

Spoont, M. R., Murdoch, M., Hodges, J., & Nugent, S. (2010). Barriers to care for veterans with PTSD. *Journal of Traumatic Stress, 23*(1), 97–101.

Steenkamp, M. M., & Litz, B. T. (2013). Psychotherapy outcome research on combat-related PTSD. *Journal of Anxiety Disorders, 27*(2), 95–102.

Steenkamp, M. M., Litz, B. T., Hoge, C. W., & Marmar, C. R. (2020). Psychotherapy for military-related PTSD: A review of clinical trials. *JAMA Psychiatry, 77*(2), 201–210.

Stein, D. J., Ipser, J. C., & Seedat, S. (2009). Pharmacotherapy for post-traumatic stress disorder. *Cochrane Database of Systematic Reviews, 2009*(1), CD002795.

Strauss, J. L., Lang, A. J., Schnurr, P. P., & Murray, L. (2011). Complementary and alternative medicine use among veterans with PTSD. *Psychological Services, 8*(3), 185–194.

Teixeira, P. J., Carraça, E. V., Markland, D., Silva, M. N., & Ryan, R. M. (2012). Exercise, physical activity, and self-determination theory: A systematic review. *International Journal of Behavioural Nutrition and Physical Activity, 9*, 78.

Thompson-Hollands, J., Marx, B. P., Lee, D. J., Resick, P. A., & Sloan, D. M. (2021). Engagement and dropout in PTSD treatment: A review. *European Journal of Psychotraumatology, 12*(1), 189–203.

Troyanskaya, M., Fitzpatrick, S., & Pfeffer, C. R. (2015). Alcohol misuse and PTSD in veterans: Clinical considerations. *Substance Use & Misuse, 50*(5), 587–597.

Van der Kolk, B. A., & Najavits, L. M. (2013). Approaches to the treatment of PTSD. *Psychiatric Annals, 43*(9), 374–379.

Varker, T., Brand, R. M., Ward, J., Terhaag, S., & Phelps, A. (2021). Emerging pharmacotherapies for PTSD. *Expert Opinion on Pharmacotherapy, 22*(1), 59–70.

Wahbeh, H., Senders, A., Neuendorf, R., & Cayton, J. (2014). Complementary and alternative medicine for posttraumatic stress disorder. *Journal of Evidence-Based Complementary & Alternative Medicine, 19*(3), 161–173.

Walker, R. S., Difede, J., Cukor, J., & Rizzo, A. (2016). Environmental triggers, startle response, and PTSD: Clinical and research perspectives. *Anxiety, Stress & Coping, 29*(6), 607–619.

Whitworth, J. W., & Ciccolo, J. T. (2016). Exercise and PTSD: A systematic review and meta-analysis. *Military Medicine, 181*(9), 856–865.

Whitworth, J. W., Ciccolo, J. T., & Nosrat, S. (2017). Exercise as an adjunct treatment for PTSD: A systematic review. *American Journal of Lifestyle Medicine, 11*(5), 408–423.

Yehuda, R. (2002). Post-traumatic stress disorder. *New England Journal of Medicine, 346*(2), 108–114.

Index

J. Alder, *Military Men, Physical Exercise, and Post-Traumatic Stress Disorder*, Palgrave Studies in Masculinity, Sport and Exercise, https://doi.org/10.1007/978-3-032-08957-1

GPSR Compliance
The European Union's (EU) General Product Safety Regulation (GPSR) is a set of rules that requires consumer products to be safe and our obligations to ensure this.

If you have any concerns about our products, you can contact us on

ProductSafety@springernature.com

In case Publisher is established outside the EU, the EU authorized representative is:

Springer Nature Customer Service Center GmbH
Europaplatz 3
69115 Heidelberg, Germany

www.ingramcontent.com/pod-product-compliance
Lightning Source LLC
Chambersburg PA
CBHW050208041225
36303CB00004B/72
* 9 7 8 3 0 3 2 0 8 9 5 6 4 *